MEDICAL ODYSSEYS

MEDICAL ODYSSEYS

*The Different and
Sometimes Unexpected
Pathways to
Twentieth-Century
Medical Discoveries*

Allen B. Weisse, M.D.

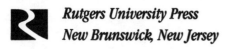

Rutgers University Press
New Brunswick, New Jersey

Two chapters, in slightly different form, have been previously published in *Hospital Practice:* "Say It Isn't 'No'" (March 15, 1986) and "On Chinese Restaurants, Prolapsed Heart Valves, and Other Medical Conundrums" (February 15, 1989).

Library of Congress Cataloging-in-Publication Data

Weisse, Allen B.
    Medical odysseys : the different and sometimes unexpected pathways
to twentieth-century medical discoveries / Allen B. Weisse.
        p.   cm.
    Includes bibliographical references.
    ISBN 0-8135-1616-1 (cloth)   ISBN 0-8135-1617-X (pbk.)
    1. Medical innovations—History.   2. Medicine—Research—History.
I. Title.
    [DNLM: 1. History of Medicine.   WZ 40 W432m]
    R850.W45   1991
    610'.9—dc20
    DNLM/DLC
    for Library of Congress   90-8387
                                                                        CIP

This book is dedicated to all the great scientists who have been recognized for having advanced the frontiers of medical knowledge—and to all the equally dedicated and hardworking men and women beside them who have not.

Contents

Acknowledgments

This book could not have been written without the cooperation of a number of individuals who either were intimately involved with the subjects under discussion or, by virtue of their own career accomplishments, were extraordinarily well qualified to comment upon them. For their participation in extended interviews and/or detailed chapter review, I am deeply indebted to: Doctors Charles P. Bailey, Baruch S. Blumberg, Howard B. Burchell, Thomas S. Chen, André Cournand, William Dock, Mary Allen Engle, David W. Fraser, Bruce Glick, Robert A. Good, Willem J. Kolff, Saul Krugman, Joseph E. McDade, William P. Murphy, Alfred M. Prince, Albert B. Sabin, Jonas Salk, Herman N. Uhley, and Paul M. Zoll.

A number of other medical scientists provided helpful information along the way, helping to eliminate errors and fill in needed gaps of information. These included: Doctors Jost Benedum, Edward J. Cafruny, W. Drukker, George J. Hill, Maurice R. Hilleman, Alan R. Hinman, Rajendra Kapila, Norman Lasker, Michel Mirowski, John F. Modlin, Christos B. Moschos, and William E. Neville.

I am especially grateful to Karen M. Reeds, science editor of Rutgers University Press, for her keen eye and helpful suggestions.

My apologies to any and all others whose "brains I picked" along the way during the six-year period involved in writing *Medical Odysseys* and whose names I have failed to mention. One whose contribution cannot ever be forgotten is Dr. Laura Weisse. Her honest and penetrating evaluations of the chapter drafts kept me on the track and off the tangents onto which my misguided enthusiasm often led me.

MEDICAL ODYSSEYS

Introduction

How Do Discoveries Happen?

In 1984 I finished a book that mainly concerned great discoverers in medicine.* No sooner had I completed this project than I felt compelled to embark on another: one about important discoveries themselves and how so many different people under different circumstances have contributed to them. As I began to tell my friends and colleagues about *Medical Odysseys* and about how important medical discoveries are made, too often I found that this would provoke a knowing smile and a nod of the head with a response such as "Oh, I get it. It's about serendipity!"

That word, once a delightful neologism, has certainly lost its sheen through overusage. Serendip is the ancient name for Ceylon. In 1754, Horace Walpole, the fourth earl of Orford and a member of Parliament, coined the word in reference to a fairy tale about three princes of Serendip who frequently made unexpected discoveries, that is, by accident. The term lay relatively dormant for more than two hundred years when suddenly it seemed to break out like an epidemic. It could be found on everyone's lips and numerous café signs. It even managed to infect an entire singing group (The Serendipity Singers). We have not yet recovered, especially in discoursing about science.

Conversations in Medicine (New York: New York University Press, 1984).

Contrary to this belief in serendipity, major advances in science are often encumbered by a lot of bad luck along the way as well.

There is also hard work and perserverence.
There is inventive daring and even touches of genius.
There are kindly, supportive, and inspiring mentors.
There are obtuse, bureaucratic martinets in positions of
    authority.
There is ambition and competition.
There is ethics and morality.
There is trust and betrayal.
There is anger and remorse.
There is generosity of spirit and spiteful jealousy.
There is money and the lack of it.
There is danger to oneself and sometimes to one's patients.
There is politics.
There are wars, which not only create new health problems
    but often serve as an impetus to the solution of old ones.

One special aspect of medical discovery relates to how many ideas there are that we think of as new but which have been introduced before, though in less fertile ground where they failed to take root. It is what I like to call the Phoenix phenomenon. An idea appears, has its day, and dies. Then, years, perhaps decades, or even centuries later, like the mythological bird, it rises from its own ashes to soar again. So it is that we often look upon a concept as completely new and novel when, in reality, it is merely the resurrection of what has gone before and been forgotten.

I recall, during my early training, an attending physician who was acutely aware of this phenomenon, and therefore, whenever some muckamuck of the medical establishment was about to give a lecture on some new great medical advance, he would hurry to the library and start searching the early literature for clues. At the conclusion of such a talk, when questions from the audience were invited, he liked nothing better than to rise and say something like, "What you have shown is very interesting, but isn't that precisely what von Helsing and Köhler reported in the *Deutche Medizinsche Wochenschrift* (German Medical Weekly) in 1878?"

Our reliance on what has gone before was probably best expressed by Sir Isaac Newton in a letter to Robert Hooke in 1675. "If I have seen further [than you and Descartes] it is by standing on the shoulders of giants."

As for the role of serendipity in science and just stumbling upon great discoveries by accident, the more mundane comment of virologist Thomas Rivers should be heeded. "You don't stumble unless you are walking. . . . There is no substitute for work in science."

The stories I have gathered in this book represent a wide range of subjects from various eras in the realm of medicine. Some have been told before, but incompletely, in my judgment. Some of the principals are gone, but, in many cases, I have been able to meet with these scientists personally, to probe for details of their discoveries, and to uncover their sources of motivation. These meetings, along with a good deal of correspondence, have provided, I believe, an important added dimension to the telling.

Dozens of books and hundreds of articles have been perused, but, to keep the narrative flowing, I have cited only major sources in the final section, Notes, for purposes of documentation and for those who might wish to read further.

Mercury Finally "Makes It"

"I was the only man in San Francisco who could treat pulmonary edema properly. You gave 'em intravenous mercury and they told all their friends that you were a miracle worker."

—William Dock, M.D.

Given the numerous potent oral diuretics ("water pills") now available, it is difficult to appreciate the impact of the mercurial diuretics introduced in the 1920s and which, for the next thirty to forty years, were to prove the mainstay in the treatment of dropsy. Dropsy was the name long given to the clinical picture of patients who, owing to congestive heart failure or certain types of liver or kidney disease, begin to retain excessive amounts of fluid, their tissues and body cavities filling up with unwanted salt and water. The new forms of mercurials, injected intramuscularly or infused intravenously, provided for the first time an effective treatment of the edematous condition, alleviating the suffering and prolonging the lives of countless patients so treated.

Beyond the realm of medicine, mercury has always had a special hold on the human imagination. Mere mention of the word evokes a host of mythological, alchemical, cultural, and scientific connotations. Perhaps it is for this reason that mercury has held a particular fascination for historians and scholars.[1]

A book on alchemy by Allison Coudert begins with the story of a twelfth-century Chinese "health fanatic" who was offered the elixir of life by his physician. As a result, he died an agonizing and slow death from mercury poisoning. In truth, much of the history of mercury, even to the present day, is associated with its toxicity and potentially lethal nature. Such aspects of its use, however, did not deter the ancient alchemists and their successors from extolling it as second only to gold itself. After all, each of the other metals had to be heated in order to liquidize, while mercury (quicksilver) was normally a liquid at room temperature.

For much of its history mercury has been associated with the treatment of syphilis. We now know that there is some scientific basis for this practice. Mercurial antiseptics have been shown to be bacteriostatic; that is, they will arrest the growth of a number of organisms. But often, following this initial inhibition, with insufficient concentrations of the chemical or inadequate periods of exposure the growth of these organisms will resume. Unfortunately, doses of mercury compounds potentially sufficient to overcome a syphilitic infection are also accompanied by severe toxic effects. The patient might survive the infection only to succumb to the treatment.

Although, in the modern world, penicillin and other safe antibiotics are very efficient against the syphilitic spirochete, at the end of the fifteenth century, when the disease was introduced into Europe, no such remedies were available. It broke out into ravaging epidemics in Europe after being carried there, perhaps, by Columbus's sailors returning from the New World.

Syphilis was named for the shepherd hero of the long poem written in 1530 by the physician Girolamo Fracastoro, who gives an account of the disease therein. The victims of syphilis in the fifteenth century and for many years thereafter turned to a number of nostrums. None of these was effective, with the possible exception of mercury, which probably did bring about a few cures without killing the patient by mercury poisoning.

The most notable of these success stories has been documented in the autobiography of the celebrated Florentine sculptor Benvenuto Cellini. In 1529 and in his twenty-ninth year, he had an extended dalliance with a servant girl-model, following which he broke out in blisters all over his body—the secondary stage of the disease. (The primary chancre or sore may be overlooked in some cases and in others may not appear at all.)[2]

Good Italian that he was, Cellini recognized that it was the "French disease" he had contracted. (The French called it the Neapolitan or Italian disease; the English and Germans sided with the Italians; the Poles blamed the Germans, the Russians the Poles, the Dutch the Spanish, and the last named, probably closest to the truth, accused the Hispañolans, as the original residents of Haiti and the Dominican Republic were then known.) An indication that informed individuals were already wary of the toxic nature of mercurials is that Cellini attempted to avoid them. He began by "taking the wood," a solution of guaiac prepared from a wood resin, a harmless but totally useless remedy. When this had no effect, he tried leeches, with a similar lack of results. Only when he began to apply mercurial ointment in the form of plasters did the lesions begin to clear.

For some, the healing of lesions signals the end of the disease; for others, it means only that the infection has become dormant, going underground only to emerge at a later date in one of its multitudinous tertiary forms. Syphilis, in its final stage, can affect practically any organ, although it shows a predilection for the central nervous and cardiovascular systems.

That this was the case with Cellini can be inferred from his increasingly bizarre behavior some time following the disappearance of his skin leasions. A careful reading of his erratic life-style during this period has suggested that the brain might have been involved, resulting in the psychiatric picture of "paresis."

It was during this time of his life that Cellini was involved in real estate dealings with some unscrupulous manipulators who, perhaps, had recognized the signs of mental illness in Cellini and decided to help it along. They invited Cellini to a sumptuous dinner including a dish in which the meat sauce had been heavily laced with mercurials. Cellini became aware of this when, soon after, he was seized with severe abdominal cramps followed by a bloody diarrhea typical of acute mercury poisoning. A physician friend confirmed the diagnosis, but, providentially, the sculptor survived this attempt on his life.

Because Cellini lived until the age of seventy-one, it can be assumed that the poisoning also served to eliminate the infection in his brain. This whole episode is memorialized in Cellini's breathtaking larger-than-life bronze sculpture of the period, *Perseus with the Head of Medusa*. At the base of the statue, helping support the mythological hero and his trophy, Cellini placed a figure of the god Mercury flanked by representations of the multibreasted venereal goddess.

Despite the adverse effects of mercury on Cellini and others similarly intoxicated by its injudicious use, it continued to be prescribed for lack of any other effective drugs for syphilis. Another factor in its popularity was its continued magical aura thanks to the pervasive influence of alchemical thinking.

Only one light appeared during the intellectual miasma of the period. It was in the person of Theophrastus Philippus Aureolus Bombastus von Hohenheim (1493–1541), and he was all of that.[3] With the exception of lust—he was never known to have slept with a woman—he had his share of the seven deadly sins. He was guilty of inordinate pride; he was a glutton and a drunkard; he had a violent temper and almost continually boiled with anger. He also happened to be a genius.

Born in Switzerland, the son of a physician, he later took the nickname Paracelsus, perhaps to signify his stature as equal to that of a celebrated Roman physician of the first-century A.D., Celsus. It is by this name that he is best remembered today. Although steeped in much of the hocus pocus characteristic of his time, Paracelsus was frequently able to shed many misconceptions in the interests of reason and the provision of good care to his patients.

In his own practice, he erased the artificial separation between "physician" and "surgeon," much to the benefit of those to whom he ministered so effectively. He was the first to describe clearly silicosis and tuberculosis in miners and dub them, in essence, occupational diseases. His views on mental illness were remarkably modern, and he described hysteria and other mental illnesses with clarity and compassion.

His conservative management of wounds and ulcers allowed for natural healing, free from the harmful interventions commonly employed by his contemporaries. Conceptually, he largely dispensed with the prevalent humoral theories about disease, seeking specific causes and specific remedies. He also clearly recognized endemic goiter for what it was: the result of inadequate minerals in the local drinking water where it was prevalent.

Not least among his accomplishments was the preparation of more rational dosages of the various chemicals that others frequently administered in toxic amounts, bringing therapeutics an important step closer to modern chemistry from alchemy. His preparation of mercury in the form of calomel (mercurous chloride) was a favored one during his own time and that of his disciples. And right into the twentieth century calomel was an ingredient of such concoctions as Guys pills, from the London hospital of the same name, which may have been used with some success despite problems with absorption and side effects.

About all this, Paracelsus later wrote and lectured in German or his Swiss-German dialect rather than Latin, much to the chagrin of the sages of the day.

It was through extensive travel that Paracelsus claimed to have perfected his knowledge. As a youth, he roamed through Scandinavia, Eastern and Southern Europe, as well as the Middle East. Although this was a common practice for eager students of that time, in Paracelsus's case one has to wonder whether his frequent change of address was encouraged by his own difficult personality.

Upon his return to Villach, Switzerland, at the age of thirty-three, he demonstrated his attitude toward the venerated teachings of previous demigods of medical practice by burning their books in front of the university in 1527. Other aspects of his personal behavior did not make such affronteries any easier to bear. Morbidly fat, he never bathed. He engaged in frequent drinking bouts with the local peasants. Although he frequently gave his services free of charge to the poor, he never hesitated to gouge the rich.

After winning the coveted post of municipal physician and professor of medicine in Basel following his successful treatment of an important personage, he lost it because of a failed suit against a high churchman who had promised Paracelsus an enormous fee and then balked at paying it. Paracelsus was forced to leave Basel and never again held an influential or official post. Although he died a pauper, his books, published posthumously, gave rise to a Paracelsian school of medicine, helping to build a bridge to the future.

Mercurials, whether used in the treatment of syphilis or other maladies, continued to have any of their benefits eclipsed by their propensity for harm either by acute poisoning or by chronic exposure. Ingestion of excessive amounts of mercury in its various medical formulations can adversely affect a number of organ systems. When taken by mouth, severe vomiting, a protective action of the gastrointestinal tract, usually occurs. If the mercurials reach the intestine, the lining can become denuded with a bloody diarrhea ensuing, as was the case with Cellini. With absorption into the bloodstream, it can reach other organs, such as the kidney and brain. Similar effects may be observed even after topical applications of mercurials.

Bichloride of mercury, until recent times, was often readily available because of its use as an antiseptic. It was successfully employed in many suicide attempts.

Occupational exposure to mercury was extremely common in the felt hat industry where mercuric nitrate was in use. Lewis Carroll's Mad Hatter in *Alice in Wonderland* was endowed with many of the attributes of chronic mercury poisoning: tremors, irritability, and mental instability. Although immortalized by Carroll (né Charles Dodson) in his Mad Hatter character, credit for the first description of mercurialism in the hat industry belongs to a New Jersey physician, J. Addison Freeman. "Hatters' shakes," which he described in 1860, was well established in Newark and its environs, where felt hatting was a major industry and where, although underreported, at least half the workers were affected to some extent.[4]

Even today, laboratory workers must be careful in their handling and disposal of mercury lest they too become prey to its damaging effects on the central nervous system. Yet all this knowledge about the hazards of mercury have not prevented the recurrence of horrific episodes of mercury poisoning, crippling or killing large segments of the populace unwittingly exposed to toxic amounts of the substance.

In recent times, following the treatment of grain with fungicides containing mercurial salts, major poisonings have occurred in such places as Pakistan, Guatamala, and especially Iraq. In Iraq in 1971, large amounts of barley and wheat seeds had been previously treated with mercurials. Despite warnings, they were planted, and in the following year the flour used to make bread resulted in more than six thousand victims of mercury intoxication, five hundred of whom died.

An equally dramatic and even more publicized example of mercury poisoning occurred during the 1950s as a result of industrial wastes in Minamata, Japan. A chemical plant emptied its mercury waste into the bay that was fished by local residents. Although only a small portion of the waste was initially in toxic form, the workings of nature insidiously led to a major disaster. Algae converted the less toxic form of mercury into deadly methylmercury, which was taken up by fish and passed through the food chain to the local inhabitants. Many deaths and severe disabilities thus occurred, and Japanese industry was forced to make some form of restitution to its victims.

Although the various toxic effects of mercury have constituted a continual part of its history, the problem of syphilis served to prolong its role in the treatment of this puzzling disease which was such a common and severe problem for centuries after its introduction to Europe. When it first appeared in the Old World, syphilis was undoubtedly more severe in its manifestations and more often fatal. With the passage of the centuries, however, it appears that, even before less toxic effective treatments were available, the severity of the illness had abated somewhat as it was passed on from one generation to another. The very nature of the disease, however, led to much confusion about its cause and natural history.

The fully developed case will begin as an ulcerating painless sore, the chancre, usually on the genitals. This disappears spontaneously, but then the spirochete multiplies in the bloodstream and as early as six weeks later breaks out in the generalized rash of secondary syphilis. Following a variable "latent period" of a year or more, tertiary syphilis will appear in one of its infinitely variable forms, capable of affecting just about any organ system. Because the disease was venereal and acquired by many pregnant women, it was often passed on to the fetus as congenital syphilis, with bone deformities, blindness, and mental retardation often the result.

What added to the confusion about the disease was that the first or second stages might be so mild as to be missed or not occur at all. (Cellini, for example, never mentions a chancre in his own account of the disease.) The third and most damaging stage of the disease might appear as the first manifestation or not at all in about one-third of those who had experienced primary or secondary syphilis. The variety and unpredictability of its forms often led to misdiagnosis ("the great mimic") and William Osler (1849–1919), the greatest physician of his day, preached to his students: "Know syphilis in all its manifestations and relations and all things clinical will be added unto you."

In 1909 an epochal discovery was made that should have put an end to the damage inflicted by mercurials, at least in connection with the treatment of syphilis. It was in that year that Paul Ehrlich discovered that an arsenical (arsphenamine or Salvarsan) would cure the disease. Yet more than twenty years later syphilis was still a scourge and distinguished physicians, usually dermatologists, were still serving in prestigious positions as professors of syphilology in renowned universities throughout the world.

Despite Salvarsan, a perusal of monographs on the treatment of syphilis written as late as the early 1930s reveals the

muddled thinking of the period between the discoveries of
Salvarsan and penicillin (which was even more effective and
certainly less toxic). One unique treatment derived from the
observation that patients with syphilis of the brain seemed to
improve if, by chance, they had contracted malaria with its
attendant high fevers. In an attempt to mimic this effect,
syphilologists took patients with neurosyphilis and injected
them with foreign proteins or even the malarial parasite itself
to induce high fevers and their intended effects in remitting
the progression of syphilis.

The introduction of Salvarsan certainly had not eliminated
the advocacy of other metallic or mineral therapies. Iodides
were deemed by one expert "invaluable" in the treatment of
late syphilis. Bismuth was another favorite, and it was often
recommended in combination with the old standby—mercurials.

Such was the status of syphilis and mercury in the First
Medical University Clinic in Vienna in 1919, where a third-
year medical student, Alfred Vogl, had been placed under the
tutelage of Dr. Paul Saxl, one of the attending physicians responsible for the running of the clinic at the time.[5]

A doctor friend of Saxl's, as a favor, had received permission to admit to his service a young girl with advanced congenital syphilis (contracted at birth from her mother) and for
whom home care had become increasingly difficult. No one
seriously believed that any treatment would, at this point, be
of any real benefit to the patient, but, in deference to his professional obligation, Saxl decided to give her a course of mercury injections. They might at least shorten her stay on the
service and make room for more pressing and more easily
managed interesting problems at the busy clinic. He assigned
Vogl the responsibility for supervising the course of treatment.

The inexperienced medical student wrote out an order for a
mercury preparation to be filled at the pharmacy for this purpose, but his prescription was for an insoluble form which was
totally inappropriate. Over the next few days treatment was
withheld while Vogl frantically pondered over some way to

extricate himself from this gaffe without Saxl finding out about it. Meanwhile the professor was becoming increasingly impatient as he passed the young girl's bedside each day only to learn that the treatment had not yet begun.

A retired army surgeon came to Vogl's rescue. Like many of his kind, he had been mustered out of the Austro-Hungarian army following the debacle of World War I and now he was spending time looking over the shoulders of the clinic physicians, trying to learn some civilian medicine so he could get back into practice. When Vogl confided his predicament to him, the kindly veteran produced a box.

"I received this sample in the mail this morning; it's a new mercurial antisyphilitic, Novasurol. Maybe you can use it. I have no patients anyway."

Vogl obtained permission to use it and began to inject the drug every other day, as prescribed. He noticed no effects of the treatment on the syphilis, but the nurses assigned to the case noticed something else.

Part of a new breed of well-educated, disciplined, and ambitious professionals, the First Clinic nurses had begun to keep highly accurate records on each patient to which they were assigned. At the foot of every bed was a chart indicating the patient's clinical course: pulse rate, respiration, temperature. Also at the foot of every bed was a large jug in which the twenty-four hour urinary collection was made and charted in bold blue each day.

Following the first day's treatment with Novasurol, the nurse noted that the patient's urinary output had climbed from its usual 200 to 500 cc to 1,200. Vogl made a mental note of this but did not comment upon it until the second and third injections, after which the patient voided daily totals of 1,400 and 2,000 cc. At this point he excitedly reported the diuretic effect of the injections to his superiors. The response was "a benevolent smile and a rather lengthly but unconvincing discussion of the wavelike rhythm of bodily functions."

As Vogl continued to squeeze the young girl dry with each subsequent dose of Novasurol, he finally succeeded in attracting some attention and a decision for further investigation.

On the same ward at the time was a large man, a cab driver with syphilitic heart disease and "waterlogged" with severe congestive heart failure. He was to serve as subject of a crucial experiment. Following the injection of Novasurol, he voided over the next day and half over ten liters of urine. "We were convinced that we had just witnessed the greatest man-made diuresis in history," Vogl later recalled. Then another heart failure patient, a young boy with rheumatic heart disease, exhibited a similar diuresis following Novasurol treatment. This new mercurial preparation was exhibiting an action on the kidney that was common to none of the other mercuruals in use for syphilis at that time.

Finally Saxl's threshold of curiosity was reached, and he and Vogl began to collect additional cases. Vogl, however, was not there for the completion of the study, having left for Berlin to complete his schooling. Another student, Robert Heilig, succeeded Vogl in this investigation, and it is he who appears as coauthor with Saxl in their landmark 1920 publication on mercurial diuretics.[6]

I learned something of this story from the cardiologist William Dock, one of my own early mentors.[7] He had spent 1924–25 at the First Clinic as part of his training. At that time it was also known as the Wenckebach Clinic in honor of its distinguished head. The Dutchman Dr. Karel E. Wenckebach had been a pioneer in many aspects of cardiac diagnosis and treatment, and had finally settled into the Vienna post as his professional home. Dock's father, himself a noted clinician, had wanted him to profit from exposure to this outstanding teacher and researcher.

Of course the mercurials were an exciting new thing in the clinic when Dock arrived, and when he returned to the United States to begin his short-lived career in the private practice of medicine before becoming an academician, he referred to the mercurials as some of the "gold nuggets" he had acquired abroad, and put them to good use. Injectable mercurials became the mainstay of diuretic therapy until the 1960s, when new potent oral agents were introduced in the treatment of water-retention problems associated with heart and kidney disease.

Like Saxl, Dock had apparently forgotten Vogl's role in the discovery, but Vogl generously has suggested that "the main credit should probably be given to the diligent nurse who, without specific orders, faithfully collected and charted the daily urinary output."

Perhaps we should all also credit good old Paracelsus, who had used his own mercurial preparation in similar patients with apparent satisfaction more than four hundred years earlier.

"Why Do They Turn Yellow?"

The Centuries-long Search for the Viruses of Hepatitis

Although hepatitis has been recognized as a human affliction for nearly five thousand years, until only a few decades ago it remained as much of a puzzle as a plague to the civilized world.[1] The keys to unlocking the solution to this particular mystery were then suddenly provided through the efforts of three men, all quite different in their interests and personalities, but all Americans, all physicians, and all alive today to relate their experiences: Saul Krugman, Alfred M. Prince, and Baruch S. Blumberg.[2]

Although nearly eighty and well over ten years past his retirement as chairman of pediatrics at New York University, Saul Krugman retains that peculiarly endearing schoolboy aura typical of so many pediatricians as seen through the eyes of other physicians. However, when he first appeared at NYU in 1946, hat in hand seeking a residency, at the age of thirty-five he was probably considered too old to start climbing the academic ladder. According to the book, in order to make your mark in medical research you have to start early and make all the right stops along the way. This applicant in no way fit the bill.

Krugman, after finishing medical school in Virginia, completed a rotating two-year internship at Brooklyn's distinctively less than preeminent Cumberland Hospital in 1941. At this point he thought it might be a good idea to undertake his required two-year stint in the armed forces. But with the attack on Pearl Harbor occurring later that year, the two-year hitch in what was then the Army Air Corps extended into five, much of it all over the Pacific Theater. ("You name an island in the Pacific, and I was there as flight surgeon!")

During his military service Krugman had seen a good deal of infectious disease, and upon his return set out to specialize in this area as it applied to pediatrics, a field fertile for such problems. However, thousands of other physician-veterans were also returning from the wars, and those who had left the prestigious teaching institutions had been promised reinstatement upon their return. There was simply no room for Krugman at NYU-Bellevue or any of the other top teaching hospitals in the New York area.

He managed to obtain a temporary position at the now defunct Willard Parker Hospital on East 15th Street. This was a communicable disease hospital to which almost every child with a potentially highly contagious disease was referred. There Krugman gained invaluable clinical experience. His application at Bellevue remained active, and one item therein proved providential. Krugman's cousin, Albert Sabin (of polio fame), had provided a brief personal recommendation. Dr. Robert Ward, who interviewed Krugman the second time around and had trained under Sabin in Cincinnati, intensified the efforts to bring Krugman on board. The result of all these efforts was the offer of an externship, a position that nominally placed Krugman within the department, but which had no provision for room, meals, uniforms, or salary. Krugman jumped at the opportunity and supported himself, his wife, and child on his meager savings from the military until a valid residency slot did become available some months later.

Ward, the laboratory man, and Krugman, the clinician, soon formed a close professional association that would last for many years. Krugman and his colleagues would make many important contributions to the control of childhood infections, among them the introduction of effective vaccines to prevent measles and German measles (rubella). But the most significant expression of this collaboration would occur at the Willowbrook State School on Staten Island, where they would confront the growing problem of infectious hepatitis.

Established in 1938 by the New York State legislature as an institution for the care of mentally retarded children, it had served temporarily during World War II as Halloran General Hospital for the army wounded returning from overseas and then reverted to its original use. In the postwar years the need of accommodations for these unfortunate children began to exceed even the most extreme estimates of state officials. Built to house a maximum of three thousand inmates, the school had four thousand by 1955, and the number would eventually climb to as many as six thousand.

In a report to the state legislature, the school's director, Dr. Jack Hammond, described the patients as "crowded together, soiling, attacking each other, abusing themselves and destroying their clothing." Beds had to be placed directly side by side with only a narrow aisle between them, making it "virtually necessary to climb over beds in order to reach children." In every respect it had become a true pesthole where severely retarded children, many incapable of toilet training or feeding themselves, bedridden and subject to seizures, were the victims of uncontrollable waves of all kinds of communicable diseases. These included parasitic infections, measles, shigellosis, respiratory illnesses, and, as became increasingly apparent, infectious hepatitis.

By the mid-1950s hepatitis was running rampant in the institution, affecting staff as well as the children they cared for. The director of Willowbrook asked Ward and Krugman to intervene in an attempt to bring the hepatitis problem, among others, under control.

An initial survey revealed the crowding conditions to be so bad that, at one point, letters were sent out to five hundred parents requesting that they consider removing their children from Willowbrook to alleviate the problem. A total of twenty-four parents replied and, of these, only two took their children back. It was clear that if any solution was to be found, it would be up to the invited "guests" from NYU alone to un-earth it.

The problem that confronted them was formidable indeed because so little was then known about viral hepatitis and much of that was probably wrong. In fact, the whole history of hepatitis was riddled with ignorance and misconceptions.

Such confusion is understandable, given the lack of knowledge about infectious diseases in general until the mid- to late nineteenth century. The visualization of bacteria and other microorganisms under the microscope uncovered only a few identifiable causes of jaundice (from *jaune*, the French word for yellow; the other term describing the characteristic color of skin and other tissues, *icterus*, is from the Greek word for the yellow-breasted martin). Viruses, although they account for the majority of liver infections and as early as 1908 were suspected by some as invisible invaders, would not be actually seen until the discovery of the electron microscope in the mid-1930s.

Lacking any real proof of a viral etiology for hepatitis, physicians succumbed to a variety of hypotheses about this type of jaundice, hypotheses made all the more convincing when put forth by scientists whose many other accomplishments have withstood the test of time.

The great German pathologist Rudolph Virchow joined others in perpetuating one myth about hepatitis when, in 1864, he reported his postmortem findings in several such patients. On examining the common bile duct, which transports bile from the liver to the first part of the small intestine, the duodenum, he found mucous plugs at the opening of the bile duct into the duodenum. This concept of catarrhal jaundice— "catarrh" signifying inflammation of a mucous membrane —related to inflammatory disease of the stomach or small intestine causing mucous plugging of the bile duct, persisted in medical teaching for generations. As late as 1942 it was retained as an entity in Osler's highly respected textbook of medicine. And for more than twenty years after its introduction for the treatment of catarrhal jaundice in 1919, the practice of passing a tube down the throats of patients to drain the duodenum of its biliary contents (transduodenal biliary drainage) was believed by many to be helpful in dislodging the mucous plugs described almost a hundred years earlier. Not until World War II, when catarrhal jaundice began to be recognized as a form of viral hepatitis, was the procedure finally abandoned.

Before then there were glimmers of light from several quarters. Certainly the emergence of microbiology led to the identification of specific organisms causing jaundice. For example, infections such as Weil's disease and relapsing fever were often accompanied by jaundice. Even in those cases without an identifiable microbe to incriminate, not all clinicians were deluded by the attractive catarrhal hypothesis. Evidence of further insights into the disorder began to creep into the medical literature.

Nothing so focuses a physician's attention on a disease as his contracting it himself. In October 1911, when a British practitioner, A. E. Cockayne, "was unfortunate enough to fall victim to the disease," he was stimulated to take a long and hard look at the problem. He subsequently pointed out important clinical differences between so-called catarrhal jaundice and entities such as Weil's disease and relapsing fever. He rejected the term "catarrhal jaundice" in the vast majority of cases and even suggested the term "infective hepatitis," postulating that a yet undiscovered microorganism was the likely cause.[3] Unfortunately, Cockayne and those physicians on the continent who shared his views formed a distinct minority. It would not be until 1939, when needle aspirates of the liver were obtained from living patients with the disease, that the primary pathology would be revealed in the liver cells rather than any "plugs."

A major problem during the first half of this century was the lack of readily available and reliable blood tests to determine the causes of jaundice in living patients presenting themselves to their physicians with this complaint. There were two major exceptions to this dearth of laboratory data so vitally needed. The first was a serum test that enabled the differentiation between two major causes of jaundice. One type of jaundice was caused by excessive destruction of red blood cells ("hemolytic" or "nonobstructive"). Another type was due to elevation of serum bilirubin, a pigment that had been processed by the liver but blocked from passing through the bile ducts and into the gut ("obstructive jaundice") either because of swollen cells or scarring within the liver itself or blockages beyond this in the biliary drainage system (e.g., gallstones or cancer).

The other major advance was the devising of a blood test that reflected destruction of the liver cells themselves, and which therefore could implicate intrinsic liver disease such as hepatitis as the cause of jaundice in a patient rather than other types of obstructive processes and hemolytic jaundice.

It was a Dutch investigator, Hijmans van den Bergh, who came up with the serum test in 1913. He had been frustrated in trying to study jaundice by analysis of stool and urine specimens. He decided to focus his attention on the bilirubin in the serum (the clear portion of the blood after blood cell removal) of jaundiced patients. For this, he turned to the diazo reaction of Ehrlich.

Paul Ehrlich (1854-1915) is remembered mainly for his development of the first effective treatment for syphilis, the "magic bullet" Salvarsan (arsphenamine). This great physician had a lifelong romance with chemistry and almost an obsession with the use of dyes for the diagnosis and treatment of various diseases. He developed a chemical cocktail, the diazo reagent, which still bears his name. He found that when he added it to the urine of various types of patients, the different colors that appeared were helpful in separating those with liver disease from those with pneumonias, from those with various infectious diseases affecting the gastrointestinal tract ("enteric fevers"), and so on.

Van den Bergh decided to attempt using the reagent on serum. On one occasion in the course of this study, van den Bergh made a procedural error. He forgot to add an initial aliquot of alcohol to the serum to make both the bilirubin and the reagent soluble in solution. To his surprise, within thirty seconds a bright pink color appeared. When he then added the forgotten alcohol, the color deepened into a red-violet hue. He had stumbled on to a way of differentiating two types of bilirubin in the serum. The first, associated with obstructive jaundice, he called "direct reacting," and the second, associated with hemolysis, he termed "indirect reacting" bilirubin. Improvements in the quantitative ability of the test were made possible by technical modifications introduced by van den Bergh and others, and the test, even today, remains very helpful in the diagnosis of jaundiced patients.

It was not until 1955 that a blood test became available to indicate the presence of liver cell damage (from viral hepatitis or any other cause). This was the procedure for measurement of serum transaminase developed by Arthur Karmen and his colleagues. The enzyme transaminase is principally contained within the liver cell, with only low levels normally detectible in the blood. With liver destruction, it leaks from the cells into the bloodstream, elevating the levels determined in the laboratory.

Although the development of reliable laboratory tests for hepatitis was painfully slow, an accumulation of epidemiological data gradually began to dispel the haze of confusion that surrounded the disease and its mimics.

By the time Krugman and his associates addressed the problem of hepatitis at Willowbrook, there was no doubt that a yet to be identified virus (or viruses) was the culprit in the vast majority of cases throughout the world. Two general clinical patterns of hepatitis were discernible: so-called infectious hepatitis and serum hepatitis. Epidemic infectious hepatitis had been recognized for centuries and had had incalculable debilitating effects when breaking out among large groups of closely quartered individuals. Its adverse effects on the conduct of major military campaigns, for example, had been recorded in detail. It was this form of hepatitis that Krugman was concerned with at Willowbrook.

The other clinical form, serum hepatitis, was a relative newcomer, having appeared on the scene only with the introduction of the widespread use of vaccination and other therapies involving the use of syringes, needles, and blood products. It

often struck with devastating consequences, the earliest recorded outbreak having occurred among Bremen shipyard
workers in 1833. After the appearance of several cases of
smallpox among them, a mass vaccination campaign was undertaken to prevent the spread of the dreaded disease. The
vaccine or materials used to administer it had been contaminated with hepatitis virus and 15 percent of those so treated
developed jaundice within several weeks or months following
this procedure. The use of arsphenamine in venereal disease
clinics to treat syphilis was soon recognized to have jaundice
result as a common side effect.

A particularly bad outbreak of serum hepatitis occurred in
World War II and served as an important stimulus to further
research on the disease. In 1942, after the inoculation of large
numbers of soldiers in the African Theater with yellow fever
vaccine, approximately 50,000 personnel came down with
jaundice and nearly one hundred deaths resulted.

There were important differences noted in the modes of
transmission of infectious hepatitis and serum hepatitis. The
first appeared to be spread via the oral-fecal route (ingestion
of the virus as a result of poor personal hygiene or through a
contaminated water supply, for example); the second clearly
seemed to be acquired by injection through the use of contaminated syringes, needles, injected medications or blood products.

Before the NYU team could make any headway in the control of hepatitis at Willowbrook, they needed to know much
more about the natural history of the disease. Furthermore,
because many of the cases were "anicteric" (without the clinically detectible telltale sign of jaundice), serial blood samples
for measurement of transaminase levels would be necessary
on a large scale.

They decided on a somewhat radical course of investigation:
they would take small groups of newly arrived patients, isolate
them in special wards, and, under close supervision, administer to them material containing the suspected virus. Behind
this decision was the knowledge that, in contrast to adults, infectious hepatitis in children was an extremely mild disease,

with mortality virtually nonexistent. While in the study ward, these children would also be insulated from a variety of other communicable diseases to which they would be exposed on the general wards. Finally, when they would be transferred to the general wards, they would be immune to hepatitis. Parental consent for this experiment was required in every case.

In the first trial, blood serum from twenty-seven hepatitis patients was pooled and cleared of any possible contaminants before being fed to eleven newly admitted patients. Ten of them developed hepatitis, six with and four without jaundice. A clearer characterization of the disease began to emerge, with one additional unexpected result. It was generally believed that, following one attack of infectious hepatitis, lasting immunity was conferred. Contrary to this expectation, Krugman found that some children were coming down with second attacks of hepatitis. Furthermore, the incubation period of the two episodes differed, one approximately thirty-five days (typical of "infectious hepatitis") and the other on the average of fifty-four days (more typical of what had been called "serum hepatitis").[4]

The serum samples from one of these children, "Mir," became the reference samples for what they termed MS-1 and MS-2 hepatitis at Willowbrook. What would later become evident was that MS-1 was really the classical infectious hepatitis infection typical among the Willowbrook children (now called hepatitis A) and MS-2 was "serum hepatitis" (hepatitis B), which for the first time was being shown to be transmissible not only by blood transfusions and poorly sterilized instruments or vaccines but at times, also by intimate personal contact. Sexual transmission of hepatitis B would later be demonstrated among homosexual men as well as heterosexuals through other types of bodily contact occurring in shared living quarters.

Perhaps one of the most important contributions of these early studies was the foresight Krugman, Ward, and their associates displayed in storing all their serum samples in the deep freeze for their own future use and that of other investigators. Alfred Prince, among others, would be especially indebted to them for this kind of assistance.

Dr. Alfred M. Prince of the New York Blood Center fulfills all the popular conceptions of what a serious scientist should look like. He is a slightly built man with an elegant, graying Edwardian beard and penetrating gaze through large, heavy-rimmed spectacles. Contrasted with this are the baggy corduroy trousers and frayed pullover knit sweater he sports within his laboratory. There is no trace in the measured, elegant discourse of the accent that must have accompanied the four-year-old refugee from Nazi Germany when he fled with his parents to the United States before the outbreak of open hostilities. He is also a gift to medical virology from a school of veterinary medicine that refused to admit the Yale philosophy major without a year on a pig farm first, a requirement declined by the candidate.

In the aftermath of the Korean conflict when the Doctors' Draft was still in effect, Prince was called to duty in 1959. At the time he was a pathology instructor at Yale working on tumor viruses, specifically the Rous sarcoma virus. The army was considerate enough to place him in a virology laboratory in Tokyo, but, as he tells it, "It was perfectly clear that the United States Army was not interested in my working on tumor viruses—especially tumor viruses in chickens."

To put his talents to more practical applications it was decided to have him work on the problem of hepatitis in the Far East among both American and Korean soldiery. Each September with disturbing regularity the incidence of the disease reached epidemic proportions, and Prince proposed that his group attempt to identify viral antigens in the blood and livers of these patients by blood testing before and during the September onslaught, right through the course of the outbreak.

Thanks to military red tape, permission for the study did not arrive until the annual September epidemic had almost run its course. Prince was inclined to give up the project, but his commanding officer and another Yale immunologist/virologist, Richard K. Gershon, persuaded him to proceed in extracting whatever information they could under the prevailing conditions. In 1962 they embarked upon a survey of 2,500 recruits, analyzing their sera for transaminase elevations, the telltale sign of liver injury.

Forty-two of these soldiers demonstrated persistent elevations of their transaminases, and four even went on to develop
cirrhosis of the liver. In thirty-two of these patients Prince and
Gershon obtained liver biopsies as well and believed they had
identified a carrier state of hepatitis where progressive liver
destruction ("chronic active hepatitis") was taking place. They
examined the liver biopsies by an immunofluorescence technique after exposure to sera from convalescent hepatitis patients as a source of antibodies later labeled with fluorescein.
Sure enough, in one-third of the chronically ill patients, what
they interpreted as an antigen/antibody complex glowed
apple-green under the microscope, with the rest of the liver
tissue providing a dark, contrasting background. (The nonresponders probably had non-A non-B hepatitis, a viral infection not yet recognized at the time.)

Prince and Gershon's enthusiasm was not shared by others
on the army team assigned to the hepatitis problem. Dr. Hans
Popper, a distinguished liver pathologist who would become
one of the grand old men of hepatology, was not convinced,
nor was Dr. W. K. Chung, then the dean among Korean specialists in liver disease. It was suggested that perhaps what
they saw on the slides was the result of parasitic infections or
immune responses to unrecognized toxins that had been ingested or autoimmune reactions of some kind. Those studying
hepatitis had been led down the garden path so many times in
the past that when a really significant finding stared them in
the face they were ill-prepared to accept it. In 1964 the paper
in the *American Journal of Hygiene* describing the findings
caused hardly a ripple.[5] "I don't think we had more than a
couple of requests for reprints worldwide," Prince somewhat
mournfully recalls.

While still in Tokyo, Prince experienced a rekindling of his
enthusiasm. An associate reported to him that, on a visit to a
Japanese Army hospital, he had been informed that, of those
soldiers who had received blood transfusions there, a full two-
thirds ultimately came down with clinical hepatitis.

"My God," Prince thought, "that's incredible! We've simply
got to study this."

With Gershon's assistance, he collected sera and liver biopsies of nearly sixty of these patients. Gershon even stayed on in Tokyo beyond his scheduled tour of duty so that the collections could be completed and taken back to Yale for storage in Prince's freezer in the pathology laboratories.

Some months later, Prince, who had since taken up a post at the Wistar Institute of the University of Pennsylvania, was able to free himself from his duties. He rushed up to New Haven with Gershon to start processing the specimens. When they opened the old freezer, the first thing to greet them was the rotting leg of a deer covered with maggots. To their horror, they realized that the freezer had been out of commission for at least a few months. As for their specimens, so painstakingly accumulated, what the heat had not destroyed had been finished off by the hydrochloric acid fumes from a tissue-dissolving experiment being conducted by the professor of pathology.

Sickened by this terrible disappointment but still undeterred, Prince decided to undertake a different type of prospective study in the United States but was turned down by both the University of Pennsylvania and Yale. He then found a home for this work at the New York Blood Center just a few blocks from Cornell-New York Hospital on the East side. Although appointed to the Cornell staff, he was not identified with any particular department and therefore given the freedom to act independently in setting up a hospitalwide post-transfusion study.

The plan, partially based on the Tokyo experience, was to collect biweekly blood sera from transfused patients and then demonstrate in those coming down with "serum hepatitis" the appearance of a viral antigen *before* the onset of the clinical illness with its attendant rise in transaminases and other liver enzymes indicating liver damage. In this way, he could answer the potential suggestion that anything he might find in the blood or liver biopsies of these patients was the *result* rather than the cause of the liver cell destruction. Furthermore, in viral infections the peak viremia (appearance of viral particles in the bloodstream) often occurs during the incubation period, with a marked fall off during the acute clinical illness when antibodies are produced. Having stored samples in advance of the clinical illness, he could maximize his chances of success in detecting the viral antigen.

At this point, the research of Prince began to converge with that of Dr. Baruch S. Blumberg, who had seen a notice of Prince's proposed investigation which invited participation of others in the scientific community. Blumberg related to Prince his own research experiences of recent years, and in the latter part of 1966 the two agreed to collaborate.

From his photographs, especially those of earlier years, Baruch Blumberg, unlike Prince, does not conform at all to the popular vision of the "research scientist." He is a middle distance runner and a squash enthusiast, and his physique reflects this. A somewhat flattened nose with closely cropped thinning hair on top, added to this physique, produce the impression of an aging middleweight. The pugillistic impression, however, is immediately dispelled in person by a warm and scholarly manner.

Blumberg, the grandson of European immigrants, began as a mathematics and physics major at Union College in Schenectady. These studies were continued by a postgraduate year at Columbia until, he says with a broad smile, "I realized I wasn't smart enough to be a physicist or mathematician, so I decided to go into medicine."

In 1950, as a third-year student at Columbia's College of Physicians and Surgeons, he had his first taste of research, one that would profoundly influence his subsequent career. As part of a special Columbia project, he elected to go to a mining community hospital in Surinam, South America. What impressed him there most of all was the different susceptibility of different racial populations to infection by a wormlike parasite, a filaria, which is the cause of elephantiasis. The residents of African origin were much more likely to become chronically affected than those from Europe or the East Indies (now Indonesia). The question why different individuals react differently in their susceptibility and response to various diseases remained with him throughout medical school and received further stimulus during two years at Oxford, where he received his Ph.D in biochemistry. It was there that "polymorphism" entered his life for good.

No account of the hepatitis B story and Blumberg's role in it fails to mention his discovery of a hepatitis viral antigen while he was studying polymorphism. Almost as universal as this mention is the ignorance of the nonspecialists one meets when the term "polymorphism" in reference to Blumberg's contribution is introduced in coversation. Yet this concept is critical to the whole understanding of what he was about and how he came to the conclusions he did. In addition, it is essential to comprehend the term if one is truly to appreciate the paradigm that the hepatitis B-Australia antigen story provides us.

Simply put, "polymorphism" refers to the concept that among different populations there exist inherited biochemical and immunological variants that may serve similar functions but that have different structures, genetically determined. One example of polymorphism involves our blood types, which may differ (A, B, O, etc.) while serving similar functions. Polymorphism may also help to distinguish different populations and account for their variability in susceptibility to different diseases, as indicated above.

To uncover such variations, there were two ways of investigation open to Blumberg: start with different diseases and look for population variabilities to them or start with a search for variation in the blood of different populations without initial reference to any disease. Blumberg elected the latter course. "If you studied variation then you would surely learn about variation."

The method he and his associates began with was, by current standards, not terribly sophisticated but extremely useful. Holes are punched in a thin sheet of gel. In the center hole is placed some serum from a patient who has received many transfusions (for example, a hemophiliac) and thus is likely to have been exposed many times to proteins not common to his or her own system. This serum serves as a source of antibodies to the specific proteins sought in the serum samples matched against it. Encircling the center well are several other holes in which are placed sera from the various subjects being screened. If there are antigens in any of the screened samples recognized by antibodies in the central well sample, a precipitate will form in the region between them.

By 1963, Blumberg and a coworker had identified one type of antigen-antibody reaction in this way, one responsible possibly for unrecognized blood transfusion reactions. They labeled it the "Ag system." To broaden this exploration for genetically determined blood protein variation, Blumberg's group tested samples collected from many worldwide locations. Then, in 1963, when testing the serum of a hemophiliac against that of an Aborigine, donated from a source Down Under, he noted a different type of precipitate develop between the two samples. The band, sensitive to differences in molecular size, was obviously different from that seen in the cases of the Ag type, and, on chemical analysis, this antigen/antibody complex proved to have less fat and more protein within it. Given the source, the antigen was named "Australia antigen (Au)."[6]

Blumberg and his group then began an intensive search among different populations to determine the prevalence of Australia antigen. It was often found to be present among the residents of tropical climates but relatively rare among Americans. It then turned up rather frequently among patients with leukemia. Three possibilities suggested themselves: the Australia antigen caused leukemia; the Australia antigen was caused by leukemia; there was another factor that resulted in increased susceptibility both to the appearance of the antigen and to leukemia.

A potentially fruitful group of patients were then studied. It was known that the incidence of leukemia was high in patients with Down's syndrome (formerly "mongolism"), a constellation of physical and mental defects related to the presence of three instead of the usual two number 21 chromosomes. When patients with Down's syndrome were studied, they indeed had a high incidence of Australia antigen. The results seemed to support the idea of some kind of genetically determined polymorphic link to Down's syndrome and leukemia. Strengthening this interpretation was the consistency of the findings in the sera of the patients with the two disorders. The patients were always either negative or positive for Australia antigen on repeated study.

The only problem with this interpretation of the data was that it was flawed. Although, as Blumberg still points out, susceptibility to persistent viral hepatitis follows a polymorphic pattern, it would ultimately be determined that what both the Down's patients and the leukemics were suffering from was not an alteration in their genetically determined serum proteins but chronic infection with the hepatitis B virus, that is, a carrier state.

Early on, certain data began to creep into Blumberg's daily notes. Among these ledgers, which now number over thirty and in which Blumberg includes many of the scientific happenings and ideas of the day, he points to entries as early as 1964 indicating that the Australia antigen was related to hepatitis. It turned out that among anemic patients with thalassemia (Mediterranean anemia) who had been transfused, there was a higher incidence of Au antigen. A patient followed for potential radiation injury converted from negative to positive for Au antigen in 1965, and it so happened that a transfusion took place in the interim. The serum of a "normal" control, a woman from Georgia, turned up with the antigen—and a history of hepatitis. Most striking of all, however, was Jimmy Bair, one of the Down's syndrome patients who was initially negative for Australia antigen but turned positive on retesting in May 1966. Blood tests and liver biopsy indicated the presence of hepatitis.

At this time Blumberg turned to Prince, among others, supplying them with this reference antigens and antibodies to investigate the relationship between hepatitis, transfusions, and the presence of Australia antigen.

The arrangement was for Prince to use a centrifugation technique at which his laboratory had developed great proficiency to separate, within different sera, protein constituents of varying molecular size. These would be correlated with the presence or absence of Australia antigen by Blumberg's group. It turned out that within a particular density band the Australia antigen could be located, and the size was consistent with that of a virus. An electron microscope was present at Blumberg's institution, the Fox Chase Cancer Center in Philadelphia, and when he later saw the micrographs, Prince was almost sure that they had found the virus he was seeking. Blumberg and his associates were much more conservative in their interpretation. What they saw they thought "could be a virus."

Prince recalls his sending a paper to Blumberg summarizing their findings and receiving back a revision that he believed had a totally different slant. In brief, Prince was convinced about the virus and Blumberg was not, and the data have never formally appeared in print. The only option was for the two men to agree to disagree and go their separate ways.[7] Despite the debate at the time, for the record both parties attribute it to the heat of the intellectual ferment and consider any controversy ended. In truth, both were wrong—and right, as subsequent events would prove. In 1970 Dane and his group in London published new illustrations of electron microscopy on sera from patients with hepatitis.[8] It turned out that the particles that Prince had interpreted as the virus were only the more numerous particles of the surface portion of the virus, the "Australia antigen." The Dane particle, present in lesser numbers but twice the size of the surface antigen, represents the complete virion.

In the meantime, additional data incriminating a viral infection appeared. One of the most striking single pieces of evidence occurred right in Blumberg's laboratory, where a technician, previously negative for Au antigen, became ill in the spring of 1967. She noticed her urine turn darker and tested herself for a rise in serum levels of both liver enzymes and Au antigen. She had hepatitis and had now become antigen positive. By 1967 Blumberg's team was able to report in the *Annals of Internal Medicine* their findings of Australia antigen in hepatitis patients as well as those with leukemia or Down's syndrome. They concluded, "Most of the disease associations could be explained by the association of Au with a virus."

In 1968 Prince also reported hitting pay dirt. A patient who was included in the New York Hospital prospective post-transfusion study and who had received multiple transfusions for a bleeding peptic ulcer developed serum hepatitis five months later. When Prince tested all the samples he had saved since the original transfusions against the reference antiserum of a hemophiliac who had received thousands of transfusions of blood or blood elements, the appearance of and rise in anti-gen titer was clearly demonstrated in the speciments obtained in the weeks *before* the onset of the clinical illness. This was typical of a viral infection and unascribable to the onset of clinical hepatitis itself. To validate his findings, he obtained coded serum specimens from Krugman and others. They sup-plied him with numbered sera they had obtained from pa-tients with typical "serum hepatitis," typical "infectious hepatitis," other forms of hepatitis, and with some normals thrown in. Only those with serum hepatitis tested positive against Prince's reference serum. To complete the circle, Prince found that the standard antigen and antibody originat-ing from Blumberg's laboratory matched his own reference standards.

Finally, from Japan came additional evidence to clinch the case that the Australia antigen really was a portion of the virus we have come to know as Hepatitis B. Once testing for Au antigen became available, the Japanese investigators evaluated donor blood samples they had saved. When the recipients of donor blood positive for Au antigen were evaluated, nearly one-fifth turned out to be positive for the antigen, demon-strating the transmissibility of the disease.

The aftermath of these breakthroughs, the application of this new knowledge to the development of a vaccine to pre-vent the disease, is no less dramatic than the discovery of the virus itself.

The first major spin-off from recognition of Australia anti-gen as a marker for hepatitis B infection was in the field of blood transfusion. It was well recognized that the risk of developing hepatitis following this procedure was approximately 10 percent.*

Of those patients contracting hepatitis B, the clinical course was predictably more difficult than with hepatitis A among children, for example. To begin with, the patients were sicker during the acute illness. Then, of every one thousand such patients admitted to the hospital, twenty-five would die from rapidly progressive ("fulminant") hepatitis. The development of chronic active hepatitis with cirrhosis of the liver and its complications was also a real threat with hepatitis B, accounting for 30 to 40 percent of all chronic liver infections in the United States, whereas with hepatitis A complete recovery is usually the rule.

By testing potential donors for Australia antigen (hereafter called hepatitis B surface antigen or HBsAg) and eliminating them, this risk could be removed. By 1969 Blumberg's laboratory had made reagents for such testing available to all those wanting them. By 1972 this procedure was incorporated as a strict regulation among all blood banks within the United States. Today, virtually all hepatitis acquired through the transfusion route is non-A, non-B.

The other major development in the hepatitis B story involved a means of preventing the disease, all the more important since no antibiotics are effective in curing it once acquired. Pooled immune globulin had been used with some success in the past. These solutions, containing protective antibodies from those who have recovered from the disease, have some value in the immediate protection of those exposed to infected blood or those with close physical contacts with hepatitis victims. But there are major shortcomings in the use of

---

*Although called "serum hepatitis" at the time and usually involving hepatitis B, it is now known that types A and B can both be transmitted in this way as well as by intimate personal contact. The same probably holds true for transfusion-related viral hepatitis that is related to neither A nor B ("non-A, non-B hepatitis") and that is currently responsible for most of the cases of posttransfusion hepatitis observed.

immune globulin: it is only 75 percent effective; it is fairly expensive; and the protection does not last long since the antibodies are gradually removed from the recipient's bloodstream. Researchers needed to find a vaccine that was safe, cheap, and guaranteed to provide prolonged protection through stimulation of the recipient's own immune system.

That this was feasible had been hinted at by work from Krugman's group at Willowbrook. They had performed a study to determine the infectivity of hepatitis B serum (their MS-2 type) after it had been boiled for only one minute. They wanted to see if the then current recommendations for prolonged boiling of instruments, and so forth, were really necessary. Their hunch about this was right, but, to their surprise, not only did injection of the heated serum appear to be noninfective, it could also be protective against subsequent exposure to the virus as well.[9]

This initial vaccine preparation was, however, crude and not consistently effective. Furthermore, the NYU team was not really geared up for the development and production of such a vaccine. Perhaps equally important was the fact that in 1970 Willowbrook ceased to admit any new patients.

Meanwhile Blumberg and his colleagues were motivated into this line of work by developments within the Johnson administration. In 1968 the government made known that it expected recipients of its largesse through research grants to make practical use of the knowledge gained and thereby provide their own future funding whenever possible. Fortunately for Blumberg, at about the time of this announcement Dr. Irving Millman, an experienced investigator in the field of vaccines at the Merck Institute, decided to join Blumberg at the Fox Chase Cancer Center in Philadelphia.

Japanese investigators had already shown that patients with antibodies to HBsAg were very resistant to the development of hepatitis if subsequently exposed accidentally to infected blood. Millman and Blumberg therefore began work on a vaccine by extracting HbsAg particles from the blood of carriers, inactivating it with formalin, and adding adjuvant, a substance that increases the activity of a vaccine. They applied to the

United States government for a patent in 1969, and it was granted in 1971.

By this time, progress on hepatitis B moved another participant of the story into action. Dr. Maurice R. Hilleman of Merck, Sharp and Dohme, an expert on vaccine development, had begun his own investigations into this area in 1968. A good friend and frequent collaborator with Krugman on other vaccines such as those for measles and rubella (German measles), Hilleman began to accelerate his efforts at Merck after learning of Krugman's heat-inactivation experiments, which provided new hope for a hepatitis B Vaccine.

The patent rights for Australia antigen, which had been obtained by Blumberg and Millman for their own institute, the Fox Chase Cancer Center, were purchased by Merck, and Hilleman felt free to move ahead.[10] By 1974 he and his associates had demonstrated in chimpanzees the safety of the vaccine they had developed. The next step was to show that it was similarly without harm in humans.

In searching for volunteers, Hilleman had to exclude laboratory workers and physicians who, either working directly with the virus or on wards exposed to patients with possible infections, were at a much higher risk than others for developing the disease. If one of these were given the vaccine and then came down with hepatitis B, it would be difficult to be sure of the source of the infection. It was decided to recruit a group of white-collar executives at Merck to test the safety of their product. Krugman and his wife, Sylvia, insisted on being included in this testing, which was carried out in 1975. The vaccine also proved to be safe in humans.

Blumberg recalls how incredibly lucky they all were in their search for a vaccine. The first thing they tried, actually the only part of the virus that had been identified, the surface antigen, was extremely effective. Theoretically, at least, one would have predicted that a more complete representation of the virus within such a vaccine would have been required. Moreover, the remarkable safety of the vaccine would be proved throughout the course of its administration.

Such revelations were, however, not immediately to be appreciated. In the late 1960s and early 1970s there were still some skeptics who persisted in questioning the relationship between the Australia antigen and clinical hepatitis. Blumberg and his group had attempted to promote vaccine field trials in Europe and had hopes that Merck would finally succeed in this effort. But it would take developments at the New York Blood Center to provide the most convincing vindication of their findings as Prince's colleague, Wolf Szmuness, took up the challenge.

Screening of potential donors for HBsAg had made all blood bank personnel aware that many individuals with no previous history of transfusions or needle sticks themselves were testing positive. In New York, with its large gay community, many of these were turning out to be homosexual men. As with the institutionalized children at Willowbrook, intimate personal contact with carriers was the obvious source, although here it was sexual rather than related to unhygienic conditions.

Szmuness, an epidemiologist, realized that for the effectiveness of the vaccine to be demonstrated in a low-risk population, perhaps as many as forty to fifty thousand subjects would be needed. Among a high-risk population, the numbers could be considerably lower to achieve statistical significance of the results. Furthermore, the trial of placebo versus vaccine (then of unknown toxicity) could be much better justified in a group at high risk. He, Dr. Cladd E. Stevens, and their associates began to look at the gay male community in New York in a systematic way.

Initial screening was begun in 1974–75. Among male homosexuals who were screened, 65 percent tested positive for HBsAg or other markers for hepatitis B infection that were now becoming available. This was ten times the frequency found in control males. There was no doubt about the risk for gay men. In the subsequent trial, nearly 1,100 homosexual men not yet positive for hepatitis B infection were randomly assigned to either a placebo or a vaccinated group.

The results of the study, released in 1980, were incontrovertible.[11] Over an eighteen- month follow-up period, clinical or subclinical infection occurred in less than 3 percent of those receiving the vaccine. The incidence among the placebo group was nearly 30 percent. Moreover, the side effects of the vaccine were shown to be minimal. The vaccine was licensed in 1981 and introduced for general use in 1982.

Many other important discoveries about viral hepatitis have followed in the wake of these initial reports. Other parts of hepatitis B have been identified, providing complete characterization of the virus. The current vaccine consists of formalin-treated surface particles obtained from blood donors. This may be replaced by other vaccines devised through the ingenious use of recombinant DNA techniques, with precise tailoring of newer vaccines to different elements within and on the surface of the virion. It has been learned, incidentally, that the surface antigen, for all its importance in showing the way toward the control of the disease, is not, in itself, infective and that other components within the virus that accompany it are the real transmitters of the infection. Hepatitis A has been identified under the electron microscope, and tests for it and its respondent antibodies within the host have been devised. Currently the major cause of transfusion-related hepatitis is non-A, non-B (so-called because of absent markers for A or B in these hepatitis patients). As recently as 1989, researchers at the California-based Chiron Corporation uncovered a new hepatitis virus, hepatitis C, which appears to be the predominant agent accounting for previously diagnosed non-A, non-B transfusion-acquired hepatitis. Also newly recognized is the delta virus, one that can exist only in the presence of hepatitis B infection. This represents a fourth category of human viral hepatitis.

The hepatitis story is, of course, replete with serendipity, starting as early as van den Bergh's stumbling onto the two types of bilirubin. Blumberg simply chanced upon the Australia antigen. And Krugman inadvertently demonstrated the protective effect of boiling infective serum. But, as one wise senior scientist has observed, "It is one thing to have your 'shins kicked' [by a valuable unexpected finding]; it's another to know when it happens and what to do about it." None of these investigators failed in that respect.

As indicated at the beginning of this book, there is a lot more to scientific discovery than serendipity or good luck. *Bad luck* plagued Prince, particularly, but did not deter him. There was a touch of genius in the decision to use hemophiliacs, those exposed to so many blood transfusions in the past, in the search for both polymorphism or past hepatitis infections. The research that went into hepatitis would surely have been impeded without the facilities such as those at Willowbrook, supplied by a state desperately seeking a solution to a problem of institutional disease, or without the federal government's financial support in building the Great Society. Later, the threatened withdrawal of this support provided the impetus for finding a vaccine to control the disease. Some competition was obviously a part of the spur to the relationship between Prince and Blumberg, although, to their credit, both have put this behind them.

Of all the participants, Blumberg has, perhaps, been the most "blessed" (the English translation of the Hebrew word *baruch*). In 1976 he shared a Nobel prize for medicine for his contributions. Interestingly enough, hepatitis was not even mentioned in the citation. It was for "discoveries concerning new mechanisms for the origin and dissemination of infectious diseases" that he was rewarded in this way.*

Blumberg, now Master of Balliol College at Oxford, admits to having been puzzled at first by this citation, but adds that, in retrospect, the Nobel Committee had been extremely perceptive in so delineating his accomplishments. After all, his discoveries about a very obvious disease arose from his findings in two individuals with no clinical evidence of it whatever: an Australian aborigine who was an asymptomatic carrier and

---

*Dr. D. Carleton Gajdusek, the corecipient, as a result of his field work in New Guinea on the mysterious neurological disease kuru, had revealed the transmission of a new "slow" virus through ritualistic cannibalism prior to the burial of victims.

a hemophiliac who simply had antibodies to previous subclinical infections.

The result of Blumberg's investigations into polymorphism certainly indicates that targeted research—a "war" on any health problem—may not always be the best way to go in the realm of scientific research.

There is an additional aspect about this particular tale that makes it especially relevant to how we apply the "cutting edge" of modern medical science. This involves the ethics of the NYU team of infecting children with the hepatitis virus in order to learn how to control it. At the time, the researchers were subjected to a good deal of vilification both from lay sources and from some quarters within the medical community itself. Even today, in the minds of some, a moral question persists.

The ethical boundaries of human experimentation are often indistinct, and it may be extremely difficult to determine where and when they have been violated. The situation at Willowbrook at the time was described here in some detail to convey the sense of urgency that gripped those immediately concerned with the overall welfare of those institutionalized children. Perhaps the position of Krugman's group can be better understood through the eloquence of Dr. Joan P. Giles, one of his collaborators. These words were written in response to criticism that appeared in the British journal, *Lancet*:

> No man has yet known absolute right or absolute wrong. We are grateful to those who would have us review, to examine our ethics. . . . A farmer may pull up corn seedlings to destroy them, or he may pull them up to set them in hills for better growing. How then does one judge the deed without the motive?
>
> Now examine the accusation that "infected material" is injected into children . . . the half-truth of the accusation is that we proceed blind and wanton for our own unspeakable advantage. The thought shames us, for here is proof that you have never known us, that you have not come the three thousand miles to know what you condemn, nor walked with us even the first mile. . . . For here is truth: you cannot clinically tell the

a

newly admitted child from the child injected, at the height of his response, from the child whose response is over, except for the fact that those who have been with us longer, by virtue of our care, are better adjusted, better nourished and more scheduled within their capabilities. And immune. . . .

Truth is many things; the truth of parents, realistic after trial; the truth of critics, idealistic and apprehensive of what they have not seen and do not know; there is the truth of those whose judgement has led to action, and the truth, acknowledged, that there are no absolutes. There is the final truth that above all else man must help man, and the knowledge that each may approach by a different path, in conscience.[12]

Into the Heart

The Surgical Treatment of Heart Disease Becomes a Reality

Theodor Billroth was not the kind of man that anyone could call a slouch. Throughout a long and brilliant career as a leading surgeon, especially at the University of Vienna (1867–94), where he headed the surgical clinic, he was responsible for a number of important innovations.[1] He was one of the first to introduce antisepsis on the Continent following Lister's lead in Great Britain. He was the first to resect the cancerous esophagus and to perform total laryngectomy for the same disease. The types of gastric resections he developed for peptic ulcer disease (Billroth I and Billroth II) remain a part of the surgical curriculum for students of medicine even today.

His talents extended well beyond the surgical ampitheater. Musically inclined from the time of his youth, he made his home in Vienna, a musical center where he often performed as second violin or viola. He was a close friend of Johannes Brahms, who was only four years his junior and who dedicated two of his string quartets to the surgeon. Indeed, in their more mature years they even came to resemble one another with their full beards and noble brows in photographic profiles.

In cardiological circles, however, his only legacy seems to have been a chance remark that has besmirched an otherwise spotless reputation. At a meeting of the Vienna Medical Society in 1881, he muttered, "No surgeon who wished to preserve the respect of his colleagues would ever attempt to suture a wound of the heart." Some revisionists doubt that he ever made the remark—it certainly never appeared in his writings. But assuming he did, and given the seemingly insurmountable obstacles to heart surgery then, one could only characterize it as wise and prudent for the time.[2]

Nevertheless, in 1896 Ludwig Rehn of Frankfurt did indeed successfully suture the heart wound of a young man and ten years later was able to compile 124 such cases in which the recovery rate was, for then, an impressive 40 percent. Still, as late as World War II, when American surgen Dwight Harken began the removal of foreign bodies (usually shell fragments) from the chests of servicemen delivered to his thoracic surgical center in Cirencester, England, the long shadow of Billroth's "dictum" marked him as a wild man in the eyes of some despite the fact that the hearts he operated upon tolerated the procedure so well. There was not a single fatality among the 134 thoracic procedures Harken performed, 68 of them directly involving either the heart chambers or the sac around the heart (the pericardium).[3]

Throughout the relatively brief but eventful history of heart surgery, the views of ultraconservative surgeons as well as medical specialists have often prevailed. On the other hand, the happy combination of an enthusiastic internist or pediatrician and a willing surgeon has proven to be instrumental in advancing the cause. The complete history of this field could fill a book, and it has, several times over.[4] The purpose here is to trace the key events that propelled us into the era of "routine" heart surgery. They are presented from the special viewpoint of one who has devoted his medical career to the treatment of heart disease.

A helpful guide to these events might be a sort of chronological skeleton I have constructed and upon which I will attempt to flesh out the whole of the story. Much of this story is often lost in the rush of telling about the rapid rise of surgery in the twentieth century. For, in truth, heart surgery is a relatively contemporary event, with many of the principals still

alive. One who is not and is often forgotten in this context is
Alexis Carrel, the extraordinary Franco-American scientist
who developed the technical bases for so many of the surgical
techniques that have become integral to cardiovascular surgery as we know it.[5]

Between 1902 and 1910, first with Dr. Charles Guthrie of
Chicago and later at the Rockefeller Institute in New York
City, he developed the technique for vascular anastomoses,
designed new instruments for such surgery, transplanted numerous organs in animals (although not the heart), and even
performed a coronary bypass operation on a dog, using a pre-
served carotid artery. Still later, in the 1930s, he also worked
on a blood perfusion pump with the aviator Charles Lind-
bergh to help support organs outside the body. Although
rarely mentioned in the routine hagiographies of cardiac surgery, Carrel's place was secured by a Nobel prize for his accomplishments in 1912.

What are the other mileposts in the development of this
field?

1905–36	Maude Abbott collects and catalogues her one thousand cases of congenital heart disease
1923	First surgical attempt to relieve mitral stenosis (Cutler and Levine)
1929	Catheterization of the human heart (Forssmann)
1930	Helen Taussig begins to refine clinical diagnosis of congenital heart disease
1937–38	Developments in angiography (Castellanos, Robb, Steinberg)
1938	Surgical ligation of a patent ductus arteriosus (Gross)
1939–45	World War II
1941–42	Human cardiac catherization is introduced by Richards and Cournand
1945	The "blue baby" operation (Blalock and Taussig)
1945–47	The establishment of closed mitral

	commissurotomy for mitral stenosis (Bailey, Harken, Brock)
1953	First successful open-heart surgery using total cardiopulmonary bypass (Gibbon)
1958	Selective coronary arteriography (Sones)
1967–68	The coronary bypass operation (Favoloro and others)
1967	Cardiac transplantation (Barnard)
1982	The artificial heart (Kolff, Jarvik, DeVries)

A museum might seem a strange place to start, but it was precisely in such a setting, the McGill Medical Museum, to which modern cardiac surgery owes part of its beginnings. In 1890 McGill produced its third class of women from its undergraduate college. Among them was a diminutive Canadian, described by Dr. Charles G. Roland as a "lady dynamo": Maude Elizabeth Abbott (1869–1940).[6] Despite being class valedictorian, Abbott was denied admission to the medical school of her beloved university, which had not yet opened its doors to women. She turned to another medical school, Bishop's College, which shared the wards of the Montreal General Hospital with the more prestigious McGill. In this way she was still able to profit from contact with the McGill teaching staff assigned there.

Graduating from Bishop's with honors in anatomy in 1894, she began a three-year sojourn at European medical centers, mainly in Vienna, where she acquired some of the tools for the work to come. By the time she had set up her practice in Montreal in 1897, she had come to the attention of some senior physicians in town and had been invited to work at the Royal Victoria Hospital. She was appointed assistant curator of the McGill Medical Museum in 1898 and then asked to assume the curatorship a year later.

The task was a formidable one, with thousands of uncatalogued neglected specimens strewn about, collecting dust during a span of over a hundred years. To assist Abbott in preparing herself for the work ahead, her superiors at McGill sent her to visit some established medical museums to observe their methods for future application in Montreal. On her way to Washington D.C. for this purpose, she stopped off in Baltimore at Johns Hopkins, where she met for the first time her idol and inspiration, William Osler.

Osler, who had begun his medical career at McGill and was well grounded in pathology, as all good internists of the day were, had donated many of the specimens in the collection. He was now in his prime at Johns Hopkins and would later become Regius Professor of Medicine at Oxford and the closest thing to a patron saint for all future internists. He encouraged Abbott and would later communicate with her about some of the unusual cardiac malformations that she had included in the collection. So impressed with Abbott's work did Osler become that in 1905 he invited her to write a section on congenital heart disease for his *System of Modern Medicine.*

Osler and Abbott's motivation during this period could only be intellectual curiosity. As late as the eighth edition of Osler's *Principles and Practice of Medicine* (1912), only four and a half of the 1,226 pages were devoted to the subject. About congenital heart disease, Osler explained, "These have only a limited clinical interest as in a large proportion of the cases the anomaly is not compatible with life and in others nothing can be done to remedy the defect or even to relieve the symptoms."

Nevertheless, Abbott persisted in collecting, cataloguing, and, equally important, divining the physiological effects of different congenital malformations. As early as 1924 she was including diagrams of the circulatory patterns of different defects and introduced a classification based on whether or not a shunting of unoxygenated blood from the right heart, bypassing the lungs, caused cyanosis (a bluish appearance of the skin) to appear at birth or to develop later or not at all. This classification is still helpful and used routinely in modern textbooks on the subject.

As the numbers of her specimens increased, she was also able to get a statistical handle on the incidence of the various defects: the holes in the heart walls between the upper and lower chambers (atrial and ventricular septal defects); blockages of valves (stenoses) or their inability to close fully (incompetency or regurgitation); reversed positions of the ventricles (transpositions), and so on. By 1936, her collection of one thousand cases formed the basis of an exhibit which was displayed in Canada, Europe, and the United States. The American Heart Association underwrote the expense of preserving this invaluable collection in printed form for all practitioners to own and learn from.[7]

The classification of cardiac malformations and understanding their effects on the circulation of the blood was a major first step. The ability to recognize them *before* they were placed on the shelves in formalin-filled bottles was the next. The pioneer in this field was another remarkable woman, Helen B. Taussig (1898–1986).[8] Physically she was the antithesis of her predecessor and later good friend, Maude Abbott. Quite tall, big boned, seemingly ungainly at times, Taussig was possessed of a quiet dignity and unwavering determination. Born in a later period and different society from Abbott's humble beginnings in the Canadian countryside, Taussig was the product of a patrician background in Boston, the daughter of Frank W. Taussig, the Henry Lee Professor of Economics at Harvard and cofounder of the Harvard School of Business Administration. She was more sensitive to the injustices of the male-dominated medical establishment, and the scars they left upon her never quite healed.* After her tragic death in an automobile accident in 1986, one of her former trainees wrote, "One cannot describe the real life of Helen Taussig without recalling the turmoil, the resentments, envy and bitterness that more than counterbalanced any recognition of her work. For many years she was under siege. . . . She suffered."

Taussig decided to study medicine in 1921. Denied admission to Harvard Medical School, she was allowed to take courses at the Harvard School of Public Health before switching to Boston University. There the dean and professor of

---

*This sensitivity may have accounted for her refusal over a four-year period to be interviewed by the author. We had finally agreed on a meeting, but her death came the week before the scheduled date.

anatomy, Alexander Begg, provided her with an ox heart and instructed her to study the muscle bundles of the organ. Two years later he encouraged Taussig to complete her studies at Johns Hopkins, where, thanks to a generous donation by heiress Mary E. Garrett, Johns Hopkins had been able to complete construction on its hospital and open its doors in 1893—with the proviso that women be accepted to the medical school on an equal basis with men.

Following her graduation from Hopkins, Taussig was denied an internship in medicine but offered a position at the Johns Hopkins Heart Station for a year. At this point, a visionary, Edwards A. Park, the new chief of pediatrics, came into her life and provided the guidance for her subsequent career. Park offered her a two-year internship in pediatrics and then, in 1930, the post as head of the cardiac clinic at the Harriet Lane Home for chronically ill children.

Taussig believed that, with rheumatic fever rampant at the time, her major task would be to concentrate on rheumatic heart disease. Like others of her time, she considered victims of congenital heart disease "hopeless finalities." For example, much in the way Osler had expressed despair, Paul Dudley White, in the 1937 edition of his textbook, twenty-five years after Osler's work, maintained a similarly gloomy outlook. Park's approach, however, was upbeat and providentially farsighted. He thought it would be no more proper for Taussig to exclude the study of congenital heart disease than it would be for a psychiatrist to exclude the study of mentally deficient children. When the new fluoroscope was wheeled into the Home to complement the other two-thirds of its armamentarium (a three-lead electrocardiography machine and Taussig), he greeted his protégé with: "Now, Dr. Taussig, you are going to learn congenital malformations of the heart. And when you do, it will be a great day."

At first, Taussig recalled, she had no great enthusiasm for such a pointless exercise, as she initially saw it. Then, gradually, she began to look upon her cases of congenital heart disease as her personal "crossword puzzles." She gained increasing proficiency in being able to predict on the basis of her clinical examination, fluoroscopy, and the electrocardiogram what would eventually be shown at the autopsy table. A particularly noteworthy day came in 1935 when she thought she could detect the absence of a functional right ventricle in a child. Others thought her diagnosis "crazy," but the pathologist proved her right, as he did again within two months' time when a similar case was presented to her. Taussig was certainly on to something. In her own words, "The key to clinical diagnosis of malformations of the heart had been turned."[9]

Meanwhile cardiac surgeons had not progressed much beyond the occasional heroic foray into the chest to suture a wound or remove a foreign body from the heart. In the 1920s Rehn and others in Europe and Dr. Edward D. Churchill in Boston had successfully removed scarred pericardium, which had prevented affected hearts from filling properly (chronic constrictive pericarditis), but what would be the next step? In the first part of this century coronary heart disease had not yet achieved its current status as a major health problem. Rheumatic heart disease was common, but, inasmuch as many of these patients could survive into the third or fourth decades of life or beyond, urgency for surgical approaches to treatment was not great enough to warrant the risks of such treatment in the infancy of thoracic surgery. Congenital heart diseases, because of the frequent death of infants and children so afflicted, seemed to represent the kind of desperate ends calling out for desperate means to prevent them.

Attempts to correct defects within the heart were out of the question, but two entities just beyond the heart itself provided an impetus for a modest beginning: the patent ductus arteriosus and coarctation of the aorta.

The circulation of the blood in the developing fetus differs from that of the normal-functioning child or adult. In the latter, following extraction of oxygen by the peripheral tissues, the partly unoxygenated blood is returned through the venous system to the right heart chambers (atrium and ventricle) and thence, via the pulmonary artery, to the lungs for

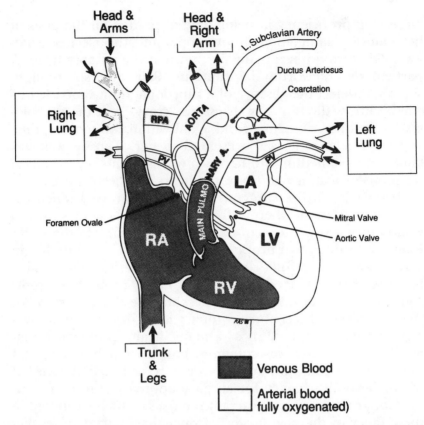

Diagrammatic representation of the heart shortly after birth, right after expansion of the lungs and normal closure of the foramen ovale, with closure of the ductus arteriosus about to begin. Unoxygenated venous blood that has returned to the heart is delivered via the pulmonary artery and its branches to the lungs for oxygenation. Fully oxygenated blood returning to the left heart via the pulmonary veins is then pumped out to the body via the aorta and its branches. In the "patient" illustrated, the usual location of a congenital abnormality, coarctation of the aorta, is shown (see text for further details). RPA, LPA = right and left pulmonary arteries; RA, RV = right atrium and ventricle; LA, LV = left atrium and ventricle; PV = pulmonary vein. For clarity, the tricuspid valve, separating the right atrium and ventricle, and the pulmonic valve separating the right ventricle and main pulmonary artery, are drawn in but not labeled.

full oxygenation and return to the left heart and out the aorta for another cycle of blood (and oxygen) distribution to the body (see accompanying figure).

In the fetus, the lungs are collapsed and nonfuctional. Oxygenated blood necessary for its development and growth is obtained from the mother via uterine vessels running from the placenta to the umbilicus of the fetus. The task for the fetus is to find some way to get all this oxygenated blood entering its right heart out to the aorta since the high resistance of a collapsed lungs permits only negligible flow through the lungs. This is done through two temporary conduits which allow this necessary shunting to occur. First, within the heart a flapped hole, the foramen ovale, permits flow from right atrium to left atrium, bypassing the lungs. Second, a tubelike structure, the ductus arteriosus, exists between the pulmonary artery and aorta so that any blood not shunting right to left at the atrial level and passing out the pulmonary artery can also reach the systemic circulation without having to traverse the lungs.

At birth, a miracle of adjustment occurs. With the first cry of the emerging infant, the lungs suddenly expand and blood begins to rush into them from the right heart. As this blood, now oxygenated by the infant itself, returns to the left atrium, the flap of the foramen ovale slams shut and within hours of birth the ductus arteriosus constricts. It ultimately forms a nonfunctioning ligamentous structure, a vestige of its intrauterine self. Rapidly, then, adjustments are made to assume the adult pattern.

The problem for some babies is that the ductus fails to close, and variable amounts of oxygenated blood in the aorta start flowing back uselessly through the ductus to the pulmonary artery and lungs. This results in a volume overloading of the heart, and early heart failure may occur in some cases. The other complication awaiting the child with the persistent ductus (PDA) is that of a bacterial infection of the structure, an endarteritis that was invariably fatal in the preantibiotic era.

However, certain aspects of this malformation made it increasingly attractive as a condition for surgical correction.[10] In the years preceding the work of Maude Abbott, it was believed that a PDA usually existed only as an accompaniment to more severe and unapproachable malformations within the heart. Thanks to Abbott, Taussig and other pediatricians following her lead, it became clear that a PDA could, with some frequently, exist as an isolated anomaly: correcting it would mean a complete cure. As for the second common complication of the PDA, infective endarteritis, for reasons still not clear, this usually did not occur before the age of ten. Therefore, although over half the children surviving infancy might subsequently die from infection, there was a golden period between five and ten when the children might be big enough to withstand the relatively crude and uninformed surgical approaches of the day and be saved the death threat of supervening infection.

As early as 1907 it had been suggested that ligation of PDAs might be possible, but it remained for a surgical resident at the Children's Hospital in Boston to successfully undertake this epochal procedure on August 26, 1938. Robert E. Gross was then thirty-three and probably first directed toward this goal by his medical school classmate, John P. Hubbard, a pediatrician at the same hospital.

Hubbard recalls calling in Gross early in 1938 to perform an abdominal exploration on a child with an acute abdominal condition in whom Hubbard, a budding pediatric cardiologist, had also diagnosed a PDA. Prior to the operation Hubbard teased Gross, "While you're in the belly, why don't you reach up and tie the ductus?"[11]

Gross visited Hubbard's cardiology clinic several times to familiarize himself with the problem and then, with the systematic thoroughness that would characterize his entire career, began his journeys to the autopsy table and dog laboratory to work out the details of the operation. By the following summer he felt prepared. He and Hubbard selected a seven-and-a-half-year-old girl without gross heart failure but with obvious limitation of activity and an enlarged heart, as shown by chest X ray. She seemed an ideal candidate.

Although, with over three decades of open heart surgery

behind us, ligation of a patent ductus now seems a relatively simple procedure, in 1938 it was a formidable and daring undertaking. Gross had been mentally fortified by the knowledge of his careful and exhaustive preparation and had also been encouraged by the support of the prominent cardiologist Dr. Paul Dudley White. He also took the precaution of scheduling another patient for the next day. Should some unforeseen complication result in disaster on the first try, he wanted to be sure to prove the feasibility of the operation before resistance to it rapidly built up.

Despite such precautions, he could not erase from his mind the story an elderly staff member had related to him in the weeks preceding the planned surgery. It concerned a bright young pediatrician who, in a child suspected of having bacterial meningitis, dared in 1922 to obtain some spinal fluid from a lumbar puncture to establish the diagnosis. Although now considered mandatory in such cases, spinal taps at the time were considered such an outrageous intrusion that the poor man was stripped of his hospital privileges, then his membership in the medical society, and finally his medical license. He had spent his remaining days in northern New England eking out a living as a chicken farmer following the ruination of his medical career.[12]

What Gross was about to attempt in 1938 was a good deal more adventurous than a simple spinal tap, and he knew his future was at stake—for better or for worse—on the basis of the result. At surgery Gross exposed the ductus, less than an inch in length and width, and passed a silk suture around it. He tightened the ligature and achieved complete success, well on his way to becoming one of the outstanding cardiac surgeons of his era.[13]

Within a year the operation was being performed by other surgeons throughout the world. It was later found that with simple ligation, the abnormal communication could reestablish itself, and complete division with tying off of the two free ends became an alternative procedure. It was also learned as the result of a last-ditch effort of repair in a critically ill patient with a bacterial infection of the ductus that, following division of the PDA, the body's inherent defense mechanisms could successfully eradicate the infection. In the preantibiotic era, such an accomplishment in an otherwise fatal complication was nothing short of miraculous.

The great success of Gross in Boston hardly went unnoticed by Helen Taussig, who on a daily basis continued to struggle with the diagnosis and management of infants and children with congenital heart disease. One type in particular, the cyanotic or "blue" babies, she found were dying early in life, and Taussig began to understand why. These were patients who, predominantly, had obstruction of flow from the right heart into the lungs (caused by a narrowed pulmonic valve, for example). Their blue appearance resulted from shunting of unoxygenated blood directly from the right heart to the left and out the aorta through holes in the walls separating the right and left heart chambers. It was a situation somewhat akin to the fetal state, only this time it was structural defects of the heart rather than collapsed lungs causing the rerouting of the venous blood.

What kept some patients alive was a patent ductus that permitted some of the poorly oxygenated blood from the aorta to pass back through the pulmonary circuit through the lungs for oxygenation. But with the passage of time, as the ductus began to close off, the children became more and more subject to a fatal decrease of oxygen in their blood. Taussig recognized that they were not dying from heart failure but, in a sense, from asphyxiation. The only way to relieve this problem was to keep the natural ductus open or create a new one surgically.

Taussig visited Gross in Boston and suggested that he begin attempts to restore such a communication in her cyanotic "blue babies," but Gross, in the first flush of success after having achieved closure of the PDAs, was not very receptive to the idea of now going on to create them. Taussig had to bide her time.

In 1941 Dr. Alfred Blalock arrived from Vanderbilt's medical school to become chief surgeon at Johns Hopkins. He was recognized as an "experienced" cardiac surgeon, having already ligated three ductuses at Vanderbilt. In the fall of 1942 he performed the first of these operations at Hopkins, with Taussig in attendance. Following the successful completion of the surgery, Taussig told him, "I stand in awe and admiration of your surgical skill—but the truly great day will come when you build a ductus for a cyanotic child, not when you close a ductus for a child who has a little too much blood going to his lungs."

Blalock acknowledged, "When that day comes, this will seem like child's play."

Such a procedure was actually not too farfetched even at that time because the technique required was closely linked to the planned repair for that other major "extracardiac" malformation, coarctation of the aorta. This defect involves a severe constriction of the main vessel emerging from the heart just beyond the point at which the main artery to the left arm (the subclavian) takes off after arteries to the right arm and head have already branched out (see Figure). As a result of this constriction, insufficient blood flow to the lower part of the body results and, more important, severe elevations of blood pressure result proximal to the obstruction, with infection, brain hemorrhages, or rupture of the aorta proximal to the coarctation often occurring. Survival beyond the age of thirty-five was a rarity.

Surgeons such as Gross and Blalock, seeking a solution to the coarctation problem, had experimented in the dog laboratory, temporarily cross clamping the aorta right below the level of the subclavian artery as they might wish to do with the coarctation patients in order to remove the constricted segment of the aorta. In almost half the dogs, however, this temporary interruption of the blood flow to the lower half of the body caused damage to the spinal cord and resulting paralysis of the lower limbs postoperatively. For fear of this complication in their patients, these surgical investigators were experimenting with interrupting the left subclavian somewhere along its length and implanting the end into the aorta beyond the level at which a coarctation existed in their patients.

Taussig vividly recalled being present while Blalock discussed this possibility with her chief, Dr. Park, and asking him, "If that is possible [for a coarctation of the aorta] why not put the left subclavian artery into the pulmonary artery? That is all that is necessary for the cyanotic child" (see figure). Blalock already had a head start on this. In 1938, while still at Vanderbilt, he and Dr. Sanford E. Levy had reported on suturing the subclavian artery to the pulmonary artery in dogs in an attempt to produce experimentally pulmonary vascular changes similar to those found among some children with congenital heart disease.

Rising to Taussig's challenge, Blalock invited her to meet with his laboratory technician to discuss the experimental approach to the problem. Two years and two hundred dogs later, Blalock was satisfied that he knew how to do the operation, although his dog model of cyanotic congenital heart disease was imperfect. He was ready to proceed.

There were major fears about this type of surgery in the kinds of patients that were in need of it. Would these desperately ill children survive general anesthesia and major chest surgery? Would they tolerate temporary occlusion of their main pulmonary artery while Blalock attempted to suture the subclavian's end into one of its major branches? Would the left arm become paralyzed or otherwise damaged as a consequence of having its major blood supply directed elsewhere?

In November 1944, Blalock performed what would come to be known as the Blalock-Taussig operation on the first of three children who would undergo the procedure over a three-month period. All survived, with none of the potential complications materializing. The first two results were satisfactory but in no way as dramatic as the third, which Taussig, present throughout, described best.

"When Dr. Blalock next released the clamps he said, 'Now I've got a beautiful thrill.'* Almost simultaneously the anesthesiologist called out, 'He's a *lovely* color now.' I walked to the head of the table and there was the child with pink cheeks and cherry red lips. The child woke up in the operating room and said, 'Is the operation over?' 'Yes,' replied Dr. Blalock. 'Well,'

*The palpable detection of blood rushing at a high velocity through a vessel and somewhat similar to the sensation to touch of a cat's purring.

said the child, 'may I get up now?' Then and there we knew the operation was a success."[14]

Although not curative, the Blalock-Taussig procedure allowed many cyanotic children to live into productive adulthood, and many would be later candidates for complete correction of their cardiac malformations when open-heart surgery became available. More than one hundred of these operations were performed annually by Blalock and his associates over the next four years, and soon other surgical centers began to join in. Worthy of note during this period is that human diagnostic cardiac catheterization had only been introduced at Bellevue Hospital by Dickinson Richards and André Cournand in 1941 and was still in its developmental stages in 1944. It certainly had yet to be widely used for adults, no less tiny children. Blalock had to rely totally on Taussig's clinical skill in almost always making the correct diagnosis, and he would operate on 150 children before a cardiac catherization laboratory had even opened at Hopkins.

Meanwhile, surgical progress was being made for that other major extracardiac malformation, coarctation of the aorta (see figure). A Swedish surgeon, Dr. Clarence Crafoord, had visited with Gross in Boston and returned to Stockholm aware of the paralysis problem in dogs and the efforts of American investigators to overcome them. Then a near surgical disaster moved him to attempt a coarctation repair in a human. During the performance of a ductal ligation in a patient, the vessel tore loose and Crafoord was forced to clamp the aorta temporarily to prevent a massive fatal hemorrhage. No harm ensued. This encouraged him in 1944 to do this electively in a coarctation patient, clamping the aorta on both sides of the obstructed segment, excising it, and rejoining the severed ends much in the way that Carrel had devised nearly half a century before.[15] Crafoord's success was duplicated by Gross in Boston six months later, and a third operation for congenital cardiovascular disease had now been established.*

---

*The reason for these patients suffering no ill effects from total interruption of aortic flow during the repair later became apparent. Unlike normal dogs, the patients, having been subjected to aortic obstruction from birth,

As encouraging as such developments in the surgical treatment for congenital malformations were, the prior experience with such an approach to acquired heart disease, specifically rheumatic heart disease, was depressing.

In terms of sheer numbers, the problem of congenital heart disease was dwarfed by that of rheumatic heart disease, which affected a significant number of individuals following a bout of rheumatic fever. An acute attack of rheumatic fever, when involving the heart as well as the joints, affects all parts of the organ—the heart muscle, the heart valves, and the sac around the heart as well. Later, over the course of years, it is the chronic inflammation and scarring of the valves, however, that is primarily responsible for the debilitating effects of the disease.

Although any valve can be affected and either become narrowed (stenotic) by scarring and unable to open properly or conversely, through loss of valve substance, become unable to close properly (regurgitant or insufficient), it was narrowing of the mitral valve orifice (mitral stenosis) between the left atrium and ventricle that was the most common lesion and the one most crying out for relief. Although these patients often survived childhood, when symptoms appeared in the second to fourth decades, they heralded an irrevocable clinical decline, with an average age at death of forty-six in the presurgical era.

It seems difficult to understand now how anyone examining a fatal case of mitral stenosis at the autopsy table could fail to appreciate the importance of the mechanical obstruction. The normal mitral opening is an area about half that formed by the thumb and forefinger in making the OK sign. In cases of advanced mitral stenosis this can be reduced to an area equal to that of the little finger's nail or even half of this. Yet the memory of heart muscle involvement in rheumatic fever persisted in the thinking of many physicians, and even so percep-

---

developed new vessels (collaterals) proximal to the coarctation. These found circuitous routes to the spinal cord and other tissues below the obstruction. Blood flow through these abnormal vessels was unaffected by intraoperative temporary clamping of the aorta to perform the repair.

tive a cardiologist as Sir James Mackenzie (1853–1925), a founder of the specialty, believed that mechanical relief of the stenosis would be ineffective. The problem of rheumatic heart disease, he believed, lay in the muscle.

From time to time others differed in their view. Another distinguished Brisith physician, Sir Thomas Lauder Brunton (1844–1916), in an article in the British journal *Lancet* in 1902 had even expressed his opinion that relief of the mechanical obstruction in mitral stenosis might be beneficial and deserved investigation. He was thoroughly criticized by many of his contemporaries for such an outlandish suggestion, but maintained his belief.

A major fear was that by forcing open a brittle valve, it might be converted to one that would not close properly, with severe mitral regurgitation the result. Such considerations did not deter Harvard surgeon Dr. Elliot Carr Cutler and his medical colleague Dr. Samuel A. Levine. They reasoned that since many patients with mild mitral regurgitation had prolonged, relatively symptom-free survivals, it would be proper to substitute this condition for severe mitral stenosis.

In 1923 they selected their first patient, a twelve-year-old girl severely disabled by mitral stenosis. Using a cutting instrument (valvulotome) blindly introduced from below, through the left ventricle, Cutler engaged the mitral valve and excised a portion of it.[16] The operation was a success but only temporary in nature. The child died four and a half years later from progression of her disease. Over the next five years, joined by the young Claude Beck, then a surgical fellow, Cutler and Levine brought an additional six cases to surgery, but all died in the early postoperative period.

Meanwhile, in 1925 at London Hospital another surgeon, Henry S. Souttar, operated on a nineteen-year-old girl, approaching the diseased valve from above through an incision in the atrium. Introducing his forefinger, Souttar manually dilated the valve successfully. Although this induced additional mitral regurgitation, the patient was improved.[17] He would be knighted for his contributions to surgery, but Souttar never again attempted the operation. Thirty-six years later, Souttar, then in his ninety-third year, supplied the answer in a letter to

Dr. Dwight Harken. "I did not repeat the operation because I could not get another case. . . . In fact it is of no use to be ahead of one's time!"

Although surgery for mitral stenosis seemed to have reached a dead end, during the 1930s and early 1940s dissatisfaction with the ineffective medical management of such cases continued to grow, and finally, within a three-month period in 1948, three surgeons independently began to achieve the positive results so evanescently suggested by those initial efforts in Boston and London.

The triumvirate included Dr. Charles P. Bailey in Philadelphia, Dr. Dwight E. Harken in Boston, and Sir Russell Brock in London. All three, using an approach similar to Souttar's, with or without the addition of a blade attached to the exploring finger to assist in opening the valve, began to report a string of surgical successes. All three are equally deserving of credit, but the accomplishments of Bailey are of particular interest, given the thrust of this book.[18]

Born and raised in Neptune, a small coastal town in New Jersey, Bailey was the son of a remarkable mother, one who had destined him to become a physician even before he was born. ("She thought that was the kind of son she should have," Bailey recalls.) By the age of twelve it had already been decided that he would make his mark in cancer research, but at that time a traumatic personal event changed the course of his professional direction.

Bailey's father, a victim of rheumatic heart disease and severe mitral stenosis, was in the final throes of his illness at the age of forty-two. As the youth watched his mother comfort her invalid husband as he repeatedly coughed up bloody sputum, Bailey decided that he would abandon cancer research and devote himself to "the much simpler job of solving the mechanical problems of valvular heart disease."

By 1945, Bailey was on the surgical staff of Hahnemann Hospital in Philadelphia and had already conducted extensive investigations both at the autopsy table and in the animal laboratory. His first two patients, operated on at Hahnemann in 1945 and 1946, died. In 1948, he attempted a third operation at Wilmington Hospital, Delaware, and postoperative complications resulted in another death. All three failures, Bailey was convinced, were due not to the operative procedure itself, but to extraneous causes that might have been avoided. But by this time he had been denied his privileges to perform any more of this surgery at Hahnemann. He knew that another failure might end for all time his efforts to continue this work.

With this in mind, he scheduled a morning case at the Philadelphia General Hospital with another procedure scheduled for the afternoon of the same day at Episcopal Hospital across town. (Recall Gross's similar strategy with the PDA ligation.) Then at the ripe old age of thirty-eight Bailey contracted measles, necessitating a month's delay of his plan. When the day of judgement did arrive, the first patient, a somewhat elderly man with far advanced disease and other medical problems, did not survive the surgery. However, the second patient, a woman with a better preoperative risk, was significantly improved. The surgical approach to the relief of mitral stenosis was assured, especially with the additional supporting data reported soon thereafter by Harken and Brock.

To this success must be added a tragic footnote. Another young surgeon, Horace Smithy of South Carolina, had been persisting with the Cutler procedure and had achieved results even superior to those of Bailey. He was present at a public medical meeting at which Bailey, the guest of honor, discussed the results of his work. Smithy rose to speak. Graciously, he made no mention of his own work other than to allude to the technique he had been using, and added that he thought Bailey's approach was the more physiological one and the method he, personally, would employ in the future.

Following the meeting, the two surgeons met to compare notes and then Smithy asked Bailey to listen to his chest. Bailey detected the unmistakable murmur of aortic stenosis. Smithy asked Bailey if he had done any work on this other, even more dangerous lesion. Bailey had not. Nor had Blalock, with whom Smithy later attempted an unsuccessful closed repair of aortic stenosis in a patient he had brought to Johns

Hopkins. Blalock was adamant in his refusal to proceed further in this uncharted surgical territory. This had been Smithy's last hope, and, less than a year after his talk with Bailey,
he was dead at the age of thirty-four.

Relief of aortic stenosis, narrowing of the valve at the origin
of the body's main artery, would have to await the development of open-heart surgery, as, indeed, would a number of
other acquired and congenital heart lesions demanding free
access to an opened, nonmoving heart whose blood flow had
been temporarily rerouted.

Many individuals contributed to the development of the
modern heart-lung machine, which permits total cardiopulmonary bypass, most notably those at the University of Minnesota and the Mayo Clinic, but none with such determination
and for so many years as Dr. John H. Gibbon, Jr.[19] His story
begins in 1931, when, as a surgical research fellow under Dr.
Edward D. Churchill at Massachusetts General Hospital, he
was assigned to observe a woman who, fifteen days following
gallbladder removal, had suffered a massive pulmonary embolism. A large blood clot had broken off from a leg vein and,
traversing the heart, had lodged itself in the lungs, obstructing
a major part of the pulmonary circulation.

The only surgical relief for this problem was that introduced by Friedrich Trendelenburg of Germany in 1908. It
involved rapid exposure and opening up of the pulmonary
artery and extraction of clots while temporarily occluding the
circulation of the heart with rubber tubing drawn tight
around the major vessels. Trendelenburg and his assistants attempted the operation a dozen times without survivors, and
although in 1924 a few reports of success appeared, in general, as one writer put it, "The basic technique he devised
stood the test of time and of repeated failure." It had never
been performed successfully in the United States at the time
this case was presented to Gibbon, and because the procedure
was considered so hazardous, Churchill elected to withhold it
unless the patient's clinical condition deteriorated to the point
of imminent death.

As Gibbon kept vigil over the critically ill woman as she remained under observation in the operating room, checking her vital signs every fifteen minutes throughout the night and into the next morning, he wondered whether such a patient could be saved if only some of the blood, now blocked from passing through the lungs, could be removed, oxygenated externally, and returned to the systemic circulation beyond the lungs and heart to supply the oxygen needs of the body.

When the patient's spontaneous respiration ceased and her blood pressure dropped precipitously, Gibbon called Churchill, who within seven minutes exposed the pulmonary artery and extracted a long blood clot—but to no avail. Nonetheless, this experience served to impel Gibbon on to a twenty-two-year quest for the solution to this problem.

Enterprising young businessmen have been known to set their sights on the boss's daughter. Gibbon did them one better. He fell in love with and married "Pete" Churchill's chief technician, Mary Hopkinson, who became not only his soulmate but his constant collaborator. Gibbon spent the next three years in Philadelphia, practicing surgery in the morning and working on various surgical problems experimentally in the laboratory in the afternoons. He did no work on the heart-lung machine during this time but thought about it constantly and, amid the general skepticism if not outright derision that his thoughts on the matter usually received, there were some words of encouragement from a few senior scientists who had earned his respect and admiration.

In 1934 Gibbon and his wife returned to Boston where he had received a fellowship at Harvard and began to grapple with the problems of total cardiopulmonary bypass. In those days, preceding the emergence of federal support for medical research, Gibbon was pretty much on his own in equipping himself for the task. He managed to purchase an air pump at a secondhand shop in downtown Boston. He constructed valves from rubber corks. He began work on cats, which were often in short supply at the laboratory, and Gibbon would often be off prowling around Beacon Hill at night with some tuna as bait and a gunnysack to catch any of the numerous strays that then infected the area.

He experimented with many anesthetic combinations, not

realizing at one point that he was in danger of causing a major explosion with one unstable mixture ("I suppose God looks after young surgical investigators as well as fools and children!"). The venous blood removed was oxygenated in a rotating cylinder and then returned through an artery in the groin, bypassing the heart and lungs much in the way it is done today. Gradually he succeeded in completely interrupting flow from the pulmonary artery to the lungs with a clamp and totally supporting the circulation of the animal externally.

Gibbon recalled their first success in this endeavor. "My wife and I threw our arms around each other and danced around the laboratory laughing and shouting 'Hooray.'"

They returned to Philadelphia and the University of Pennsylvania in 1936, but World War II interferred with the work until 1946. They then expanded the circulatory capacity of the apparatus so that now dogs could be bypassed. They then received a vitally needed grant and technical assistance from IBM for the design and construction of equipment that could be used in humans. Following an initial failure in a year-old infant, Gibbon finally triumphed on May 6, 1953, when he performed the first successful complete cardiopulmonary bypass (twenty-six minutes) in an eighteen-year-old girl, with closure of a large hole between the upper chambers of the heart (atrial septal defect).

The ability to operate in a bloodless field and on a nonmoving "target" after elective cardiac arrest was introduced allowed Gibbon and other emerging cardiac surgeons to correct additional congenital defects within the heart, to insert prosthetic valves after removal of those damaged irreparably by disease, and later to perform coronary artery bypass operations. Curiously, pulmonary embolism, the condition that led Gibbon to this line of research in the first place, is rarely the indication for cardiopulmonary bypass today. Although the cause of death in many patients, it is often unrecognized clinically; and when an acute massive pulmonary embolism *is* recognized premorten, in those patients likely to succumb, death often occurs before proper surgical relief can be instituted.

What of the other milestones I have listed?

The technique of cardiac catheterization was vital to the progress of heart surgery because it enabled cardiologists to make more precise diagnoses for their surgical colleagues. The safety of passing a catheter into an arm or leg vein of a patient and advancing it into the heart was seriously questioned until 1929, when Werner Forssmann, then a twenty-five-year-old surgical house officer in Eberswalde, near Berlin, performed the procedure on himself repeatedly after a first attempt which he documented by then climbing several flights of stairs to the X-ray department to demonstrate the presence of the catheter tip lying harmlessly in his right atrium. But when he later went to work for the great Ernst Sauerbruch at the Charité Hospital in Berlin, his chief greeted his request to pursue this with "I'm running a clinic here, not a circus."

Forssmann's goal was to demonstrate that when cardiac emergencies occurred, lifesaving drugs could be administered quickly and effectively through this route rather than by blindly inserting a long needle through the chest wall and into the heart and risking damage to the heart and other structures along the way. It remained for two New York physicians, Dickinson Richards and André Cournand to open up the diagnostic possibilities of this procedure.[20]

Richards and Cournand were primarily interested in pulmonary diseases such as tuberculosis and emphysema and their relation to cardiac function. To do this research, they needed to measure cardiac output. And to measure cardiac output accurately, they needed a venous blood sample that represented an average of all the blood returning to the heart from various parts of the body (arms, legs, liver, kidney, brain, etc.), the oxygen concentrations of which could vary widely. Only samples from the right heart itself could provide them with accurate reflections of "mixed venous" oxygen concentration for such determinations.

By developing the technique of cardiac catheterization in 1941, they would succeed in accomplishing this goal. From this work, the ability to diagnose accurately a variety of congenital and acquired heart conditions naturally derived. But, given the traditional resistance to such an invasive procedure, it might not have caught on if it were not for the advent of Pearl Harbor and the beginning of World War II for the United States.

The military medical authorities knew from past experience that wound-related shock would be a major problem and had appointed Dr. Alfred Blalock of Johns Hopkins and the "blue baby" operation to head the Shock Committee. Cournand approached Blalock and indicated how useful the procedure of cardiac catheterization might be in the study of such a condition. Shortly after, Cournand and Richards received federal support and permission to study a wide variety of shocklike states in humans. The safety of human cardiac catheterization was soon established.

Even before the studies of Cournand and Richards, a Cuban pediatrician, Augustin W. Castellanos, reported in 1937 that by injecting radiopaque media through a peripheral vein in children, certain congenital cardiac defects could be demonstrated on X-ray film. In the following year Drs. George P. Robb and Israel Steinberg of New York improved upon this technique. In subsequent years these peripheral injections were supplanted by central injections, which gave better definition to the underlying anatomy, and cardiac angiography was incorporated as an integral part of diagnostic cardiac catheterization.

As rheumatic valvular disease began to be replaced by coronary heart disease as the primary cardiac problem among American citizens, the need to identify the location and severity of coronary artery obstructions became pressing. Selective coronary arteriography, the direct introduction of radiopaque material into the origins of the coronary arteries with motion pictures outlining the anatomy, was introduced by Dr. F. Mason Sones at the Cleveland Clinic in the late 1950s and early 1960s. His surgical associates, primarily Drs. René Favoloro and Donald B. Effler, found that such occlusions or narrowings could be bypassed by strips of leg veins hooked up to the aorta at one end and beyond the lesions at the other. The veins held up exceedingly well, and the "cabbage" operation (CABG, coronary artery bypass grafting) became the standard approach for the surgical treatment of this disease.

End-stage heart disease, not amenable to either coronary bypass procedures or valve replacement, remained the final frontier for the cardiac surgeon. Diseases affecting the heart muscle directly (cardiomyopathies), and often occurring in relatively young individuals, required a different approach. A major attempted solution in such instances has been cardiac transplantation. This was first achieved in a human patient by Dr. Christiaan Barnard in Capetown in 1967 and continued in a major way at Stanford by his fellow alumnus from the University of Minnesota surgical program, Norman E. Shumway. Another approach, given the large number of potential candidates without available donor hearts, has been the artificial heart, introduced at the University of Utah in 1982 by Drs. Robert K. Jarvik, William DeVries, and Willem J. Kolff. The application of this revolutionary new development in the treatment of advanced heart disease still faces an uncertain future.

Such, to one observer, are the major turning points in the progression of twentieth-century heart surgery. If these are to be considered the highlights, what other critical elements might be concealed in the metaphorical shadows?

In regard to this, a 1974 article authored by Drs. Julius H. Comroe and Robert D. Dripps and entitled "Ben Franklin and Open Heart Surgery" has become something of a classic.[21] It was written in response to a growing belief in Washington, D.C., the major source of research support, a belief most clearly enunciated in an earlier speech by Lyndon Johnson. As president in 1966, he expressed the view that perhaps the national research effort had been misdirected and that there was a need for presidents "to show more interest in what the specific results of research are in their lifetime, and in their administration." Johnson stressed that a good deal of basic research had been done and that the emphasis would better be placed on what came to be known as targeted research. He concluded that *"We must be sure that no life-saving discovery is locked up in the laboratory"* (italics added).

To indicate the fallacy in this kind of thinking, Comroe and Dripps took the development of cardiac surgery as *the* most dramatic achievement in the post-World War II years. The thrust of their argument was that this achievement was made possible only through the culmination of efforts by many workers in many branches of medical science. To illustrate this point, they had drawn a figure of a medical Mount Everest as viewed from the front and standing atop it, scalpel in his hand, the conquering cardiac surgeon. In a second figure, the view from the rear was quite different. From this vantage point, it was seen that there was no great single leap to the top bur rather, chiseled steplike up the mountain, there were the contributions of anatomy, chemistry, microscopy, physics, electronics, microbiology, hematology, radiology, and so on, without which the modern era of cardiac surgery would never have arrived.

What I have attempted here is to extend this concept, linking up the contributions along the way that have helped make the ascension possible. While it is fitting that the cardiac surgeon is often pictured as a male, strong and decisive—they often are—of all the branches of medicine, the surgical specialties have been the least yielding in their acceptance of women. It is therefore all the more ironic that the foundations of cardiac surgery, perhaps the most elite of all, were in large part laid by nonsurgeons and especially by two women whose entrance into medicine itself was so difficult, tentative, and ultimately so unexpectedly rewarding.

The Long Pause

The Discovery and Rediscovery of Penicillin

"That's funny."

The young physician cleaning up his laboratory noticed an unusual finding on the culture plate he was about to discard. There was something compelling about it, something that transfixed him and prevented him from tossing it on the pile of other plates that would soon find their way into the daily garbage at St. Mary's Hospital in London on that morning in the fall of 1928.

He had streaked the culture plate with staphylococci a few weeks earlier and now noted that near one edge of the plate a contaminant mold was growing. In the area surrounding the mold the staph colonies were translucent and smaller than the more robust snowy white normal colonies growing farther away from the mold. Something was coming from the mold that was actually destroying the disease causing bacteria in the vicinity.

The mold was *Penicillium,* the substance it produced penicillin, and the discoverer was Alexander Fleming. He soon found penicillin effective against other bacteria responsible for widespread human disease and death, and Fleming became intrigued by the possibility this suggested for the effective treatment of such diseases. However, neither his presentations at scientific meetings nor his publications on penicillin lit the spark. The work would lie fallow for twelve years before being once again taken up by others who would vindicate both penicillin and Fleming.

This is the popular legend about penicillin and its discoverer that has come down to us through the years. Usually forgotten in this history are the contributions of the Oxford group which included Howard Florey, Ernst Chain, and others, even though Florey and Chain would deservedly share the Nobel prize awarded to Fleming in 1945. Also generally forgotten are the ill feelings engendered by the publicity attending the release of penicillin in the 1940s, publicity that generally excluded the Oxford investigators in favor of Fleming, who had all but ignored his own incompleted discovery for over a decade. Finally, there have remained a number of inconsistencies regarding the "myth" that have awaited adequate explanations.

Now, over a half century since that fateful September day when Fleming almost destroyed the evidence of his own discovery, the dust has finally settled thanks mainly to the recent works of two Britons. Professor Gwyn MacFarlane, an Oxford pathologist, has published new biographies of both Fleming and Florey.[1] Professor Ronald Hare, a bacteriologist at St. Mary's Hospital during the time of Fleming's preeminence, has provided additional sleuthing to explain many of the seeming inconsistencies of the penicillin story.[2]

Alexander Fleming was born in Scotland in 1881. His father died when Alex was seven, and at the age of fourteen the boy moved to London to live with his older brother, Tom, a medical doctor specializing in ophthalmology. For the first four years in London Fleming was employed in a shipping office, which was to prove of little interest or challenge to the clever young Scot. The death of a bachelor uncle and a legacy of £ 250 provided him with an escape from the drudgery of this employment. He decided to pursue a career in medicine.

Nearly twenty by the time he applied to medical school, Fleming had not had any formal schooling since the age of sixteen. He also lacked the necessary Latin included in the examinations he would have to take to enter a London medical school. He studied on his own, hired a Latin tutor, and passed with honors. Among all the schools he could have chosen, he selected St. Mary's—only because it was within the shortest walking distance from his home. He entered in 1901 and would remain there as a student and then staff member for the next fifty-one years, the whole of his professional life.

If one had to characterize the four sides to the cornerstone of Fleming's career leading to penicillin, the following might well be identified: Sir Almroth Wright, syphilis, World War I, and a curious substance he came to call lysozyme.

Sir Almroth Wright had been professor of pathology at St. Mary's since 1902. Owing to a double vacancy at the time he assumed this responsibility, Wright was also in charge of bacteriology when Fleming arrived at the school. Wright would remain in charge of the bacteriology department as Fleming's superior until his retirement at the age of eighty-five in 1946, a year after Fleming won the Nobel prize in medicine.

Wright was one of those glorious British monstrosities, the kind of brilliant eccentric for which English society has always provided such fertile ground. Physically he was enormous in height and bulk, a "bear of a man," with a blinding intellect and an ego to match. In addition to his scientific background, he was a classical scholar who spoke seven languages, read eleven, and had committed to memory many thousands of lines of verse on which he often loved to test his audience. No wonder his enemies took delight in calling him "Almost Wright" whenever they had the chance.

He had received most of his early scientific training on the Continent when, only a few years earlier, the monumental achievements of Pasteur and Koch had demonstrated the bacterial nature of so many of the diseases that accounted for the disability and deaths of the populace. In the absence of effective chemotherapeutic agents in these early years, Wright devoted his efforts to the prevention or treatment of these diseases by enhancing the body's natural protective barriers to infection.

To prevent or minimize in advance the effects of exposure

to certain diseases, protection against the offending agent could be induced by *active immunization*, the introduction of a mild or modified form of the bacterium that would stimulate the production of antibodies to provide future protection. This technique, of course, was the basis for Edward Jenner's (1749–1823) use of vaccination: injecting under the skin of a susceptible individual a small amount of fluid from the pustule of the mild disease cowpox (*vacca* is the Latin word for "cow") to confer future protection against the ravages of smallpox during ensuing epidemics.

Another approach to such therapy involved *passive immunization*—the transfer to patients of previously produced antibodies to bacteria or their poisonous products (toxins) after the patient had been exposed to the disease and had no previous protection. The source of such antibodies would usually be the serum of an animal, such as a horse. Although antibiotics have become the mainstay in the treatment of most bacterial diseases, immunization is still employed in the control of many viral diseases because of the resistance by these smaller infective particles to most currently available antibiotics.

Some of Wright's earliest experiences were with the British military in India and then in South Africa during the Boer War when he unsuccessfully attempted to introduce such preventive medicine to control potential outbreaks of typhoid fever. Wright was, of course, correct in his thinking but unable to convince the skeptical authorities. When giving evidence before a military tribunal, he was asked if he had anything more to say. His response was typical. "No, sir. I have given you the facts. I can't give you brains." Needless to say, the top brass were happy to see him out of the service and on his way to St. Mary's when the time came.

At his new post in London, Wright gathered about him a group of young physicians who, in awe of and inspired by him, began to establish a proper setting for clinical research of infectious diseases. A special component of this was the Inoculation Department, set up by Wright in 1907 for the production and sale of a number of vaccines for a variety of illnesses ranging from acne to pneumonia.

By the end of 1906, Fleming had passed all his medical examinations with distinction and was on his way to becoming a surgeon. He was, however, persuaded to stay on at St. Mary's and work for an advanced degree when an opening occurred in Wright's department. The deciding factor in this critical turn of Fleming's career was, of all things, the desire of St. Mary's to keep the sharpshooting Fleming on the hospital's rifle team, which was in the running for a prestigious cup.

Among all the young men working for Wright, Fleming must have provided the most contrast to his chief. Despite his physical prowess and a slightly pugnacious look, thanks to a broken nose resulting from an accidental collision with a classmate as a boy, Fleming was both slim and diminutive, under five feet, six inches. He was also, especially during these early years, on the reticent side, although possessed of a quiet kind of wit. He nonetheless managed to distinguish himself by demonstrating an ingenuity in experimental techniques that became his hallmark. He was one of the few who could say no to Sir Almroth and make it stick without getting fired.

During these initial years with Wright, Fleming still felt himself headed toward a career in surgery and even passed the examination to become an FRCS (Fellow, Royal College of Surgeons). But then, in 1910, came Salvarsan.

Paul Ehrlich, the German successor to Koch in the field of microbiology, had begun to recognize the limitations of serum therapy in many infectious diseases, especially those caused by larger unicellular organisms such as the protozoa. Classified among these was one responsible for the most ravaging of human afflictions, the spiral-shaped *Treponema pallidum* which was the cause of syphilis.

After systematically testing hundreds of chemical substances that might kill this organism without doing harm to the patient, Ehrlich, on the six hundred and sixth try, succeeded in finding his "magic bullet," the arsenical preparation #606 which was later named Salvarsan. Wright, a personal friend of Ehrlich, was one of the first in England to receive a supply of the drug and put Fleming in charge of the program at St. Mary's since he had already been working on an improvement on the Wasserman Test for the serological diagnosis of the disease.

Not only was this a boost to Fleming's reputation, but, undoubtedly, it must have driven home to him the fact that the immunological approach to the treatment of infectious disease might not be the only one.

Soon thereafter the First World War broke out. Wright, Fleming, and others of their group were assigned to Boulogne in France to establish a unit for the treatment and investigation of war wound infections pouring in from the front. Up to this time *antisepsis,* as introduced by Sir Joseph Lister (1827–1912), was the standard treatment in wound surgery. Dilute carbolic acid was introduced into the contaminated tissues and also used to disinfect the surgeon's hands. Eventually, such an approach both in the civilian setting and in regard to war wounds would be supplanted by the practice of *asepsis,* the scrubbing of the surgeon's hands *before* the operation and the use of sterile instruments and drapes in surgery. Although recommended years before antisepsis by the Hungarian obstetrician Ignaz Semmelweiss for the prevention of childbed (puerperal) fever in women, asepsis only gradually became adopted years after Semmelweiss's own tragic death in 1865.

Meanwhile, just behind the front lines in Boulogne, Wright, Fleming, and their associates soon found that the traditional use of antiseptic methods was having little effect on controlling the infections so often complicating the wounds they examined. They conclusively demonstrated that the antiseptics were not reaching the many hidden recesses of the jagged war wounds where organisms such as those causing gas gangrene could flourish. They also showed that the properties of the antiseptics themselves were in part responsible for their therapeutic failures because in addition to destroying bacteria, they were found to kill off the white blood cells, the body's natural defense mechanism for handling microbial intruders.

They advised irrigation of the wounds with physiological salt solution which was similar to the body's natural liquid medium. This washing out of the wound of contaminating bacteria along with "debridement," the trimming away of dead tissue around the edges of the wounds, would prove to be the most effective treatment until the introduction of less harmful chemotherapy became available. Fleming published a dozen papers concerning this work in Boulogne and gained recognition as an expert in war wounds. He must also have recognized that not only would any future antimicrobial agent have to be effective against bacteria; it would also have to be gentle enough to be tolerated by the patient's tissues. Significantly, in his Nobel address some twenty years later, Fleming would describe his studies on antiseptics and the white cells as "probably the best experiment I ever did."

The final vital element in Fleming's preparation for penicillin undoubtedly began in 1921 with the lysozyme work, which, in so many ways, was a dress rehearsal for penicillin. The beginning was similarly accidental. For reasons still not clear, Fleming decided to take some mucus discharge from his nose, dilute it in saline, and add a drop to each of three previously streaked bacterial solutions before incubating them for eighteen hours. One of the bacteria, a coccus (spherically shaped organism) from his own nose, was unable to grow in the area of the mucus drop, although the other two types of bacteria did. Obviously something in the mucus prevented at least one type of bacterium from growing, and Fleming set out to determine whether any other bodily secretions had the same action and what other microorganisms might be similarly inhibited.

Fleming found that tears, saliva, and blood also had this effect on his "A.F. coccus," but that, unfortunately, when tested on a number of well-known pathogenic bacteria, the substance was of no use. Still, Fleming suspected it to be a clue to the body's protective mechanisms and to be an enzyme, although it would be left to others to finally demonstrate this to be so. Fleming called the substance "lysozyme" to reflect its probable structure and its lytic (bacterial-dissolving) action.

Although the lysozyme work proved a dead end in practical terms at the time, Fleming thought it sufficiently important to

present before the Medical Research Club which had been or-
ganized by Wright for the purpose of sharing such scientific
knowledge. The presentation caused hardly a ripple.

The next significant event in Fleming's career was the discovery of penicillin in September of 1928. The story that has
generally been accepted—and perpetuated by Fleming's own
accounts—was that, on examining a plate on which he had
previously cultured staphylococci, he found it had been contaminated with a mold, later identified as *Penicillium,* and that
in an area surrounding the mold the staph colonies were obviously being destroyed by something coming from the mold.
The source of the mold was widely believed to be the outside
neighborhood from which it entered through an open window
in Fleming's lab. This story, after one sifts through the evidence that has come to light in recent years, turns out to be
only partly true, with the real facts revealing an accident of
fate even more incredibly serendipitous than previously believed.

As brilliant an experimentalist as he was, Fleming was not
the neatest of laboratory workers. On that September morning he had just returned from a vacation and began to clean
up the mess of plates that he had cultured prior to his departure and which still remained on the bench. The plate in question had apparently already been tossed with some others into
a tray of lysol. As Fleming continued his cleanup, an assistant,
Merlin Pryce, stopped by, and Fleming began to show him
some of the plates he was discarding. Miraculously, the plate
with the *Penicillium* contaminant, although in the disinfectant
tray, rested on some others and had not been submerged.
Fleming retrieved it to show to Pryce. It was at this point he
noted the phenomenon described, murmured, "That's
funny," and held on to the plate to show others. This was the
beginning.[3]

The source of the mold has come into question. A number
of workers at St. Mary's at the time have indicated that the
window in question was never opened. They did not want culture plates falling on the heads of passing pedestrians. They
finally concluded that in all likelihood the mold originated

from the mycology laboratory one floor below, where Dr. C. J. LaTouche was working. It was LaTouche who identified the mold as *Penicillium* for Fleming and who, when checking it against other samples in his own laboratory, found a sample identical in just about every way to Fleming's. Equally fortuitous was this particular strain of *Penicillium notatum*. In subsequent years hundreds of *Penicilliums* would be tested for antibacterial activity, and the contaminant of Fleming's staph plate would turn out to be one of the three most effective.

Even more extraordinary than the above were the circumstances leading to the phenomenon that Fleming chanced upon. When later workers tried to repeat the experiment of adding *Penicillium* to existing staph cultures, they were unsuccessful. The reason for this was not really appreciated until 1940, when Dr. A. D. Gardner, an Oxford bacteriologist, carefully observed the effect of penicillin under the microscope. Penicillin was effective against these organisms only when they were actively in the stage of division. Mature bacteria were resistant to dissolution or lysis. How, then, can one explain Fleming's initial discovery?

Professor Ronald Hare has come up with an ingenious theory that could account for the success of Fleming's initial mold and the failure of those who thought they were duplicating the experiment. By tracing Fleming's activities during the summer of 1928 and checking them against the climatic conditions of London at that time, he deduced that the mold growth actually must have occurred *before* that of the staphylococci rather than following it. In the days immediately following the time of Fleming's planting the staph on the culture plate, an unusually cold spell occurred during which conditions were quite unfavorable for the growth of these bacteria. It is likely that during this time the contamination with *Penicillium* occurred, and the mold began to produce its antibacterial products. In the ensuing warmer weather, when prevailing temperatures became favorable for the growth of the staph cultures, penicillin was already present on the plate to prevent the spread of staph wherever it had diffused.

Fleming's next job was to test the mold against a number of

other bacteria. Unlike the case with lysozyme, he found that it was effective against many of the microorganisms responsible for common and deadly human diseases. After the bacteriologist LaTouche had identified the mold as a *Penicillium*, Fleming soon replaced his original term for the active substance, "mold juice," with "penicillin."

Of equal importance to penicillin's range of activity against bacterial pathogens was the fact that, unlike the antiseptics Fleming had studied in World War I, penicillin did not have any adverse effects on the body's natural protectors, the white blood cells. Several injections into rabbits and mice also indicated its harmlessness.

Given these excellent attributes, why was the penicillin work not pursued to its logical conclusion as a therapeutic agent? The traditional lore includes Fleming's lackluster oratorical style before the medical conferences at which he presented his data; the lack of sufficient resources in terms of laboratory funds and chemists to help him with purifying and increasing the potency of his preparations; lack of patient material; and finally even professional jealousy and obstructionism. The real reasons, in retrospect, are quite different and perfectly logical.

Early on, some potential problems became apparent. First, Fleming found that whereas chemical antiseptics killed bacteria within a few minutes in laboratory preparations, penicillin required from two to four hours to have a similar effect. Second, when penicillin was combined with whole blood or serum, it tended to lose its potency, suggesting that in wounds with large amounts of pus and other blood products it might be inactivated. Third, after injection into an ear vein of a rabbit and with blood samples taken periodically thereafter for testing, it was found that penicillin was rapidly removed from the bloodstream: samples taken at thirty minutes were almost completely devoid of activity.

Of what use might be an antibacterial agent that took several hours to act but was removed from the body within thirty minutes and inhibited by the blood with which it would obviously be mixing? Such considerations plus a few tentative unsuccessful animal experiments, too few in number and faulty in design, discouraged further trials. The only hopeful aspects of this early work were the possibilities that penicillin might be helpful in superficial local infections and that it might assist in the laboratory isolation of certain resistant bacteria by preventing overgrowth on the culture plate of the sensitive organisms which might otherwise crowd them out. In Fleming's landmark paper that appeared in the *British Journal of Experimental Pathology* in 1929, this laboratory quirk was highlighted much more than penicillin's possible use as a clinical agent.[4] At the time, a bacillus (rod-shaped organism) was believed to be the cause of influenza,* and penicillin added to culture material proved helpful in isolating it.

One might well wonder why, given the uncontrolled devastation of bacterial diseases upon the population of the time, no further experiments on animals or humans were undertaken. The rapid disappearance of penicillin from the blood has already been mentioned. In contrast, it was already established that one dose of Salvarsan was still in the blood for as long as six hours and believed effective in treating syphilis because of this persistence for several days. This and the other potential shortcomings of penicillin must have weighed on Fleming's mind. Even the choice not to use animal experiments more extensively, a routine practice of investigators on the Continent, could be defended by Fleming and his group. After all, there might be differences between humans and other animals in resistance or susceptibility to different infections. Finally, the St. Mary's group were committed to the *in vitro* slide and test tube methods that had served them so well in the past. They could see no reason for doubting the reliability of what such studies told them about penicillin.

Between 1929 and 1942 Fleming published only one more paper on penicillin, one concerning its use in the selective culturing of certain bacteria. Even in 1935, when sulfonamides were introduced from Germany and recognized worldwide as effective chemotherapy, rather than being drawn back to penicillin, Fleming and his group urged combination therapy with

*A virus was later found to be the true etiological agent.

sulfonamides and vaccines to treat infection. The final emergence of penicillin would have to await Howard Florey, Ernst Chain, and their collaborators at Oxford at the outbreak of the Second World War.

As with the case with Wright, Howard Walker Florey presented another study of contrasts when his background and personality were compared with that of his predecessor. Fleming, the small, reserved Scot, was, nontheless, apparently at ease with himself and confident in his innate abilities. He was content to remain at St. Mary's in the shadow of Wright for almost his entire career. Florey, the brash Australian, was constantly, it appears, striving to prove himself and driven toward professional advancement by frequent changes of position.

Much of this may be related to their national backgrounds. The English have always had a grudging admiration for the Scots' industry and intelligence. In medicine, especially, the Universities of Glasgow and Edinburgh were recognized as centers of learning for decades before their English counterparts had distinguished themselves. The "Aussies" were another story. Although Florey came from a comfortable family background, Australia was still looked upon very much as a colony—and originally a penal colony at that. The Australians' grating "Limey" accent was, no doubt, another reminder of this past and something of an impediment in the class-conscious British society of the time.

Florey graduated from the medical school in Adelaide in 1921 and came to Oxford on a Rhodes Scholarship. This later led to positions at Cambridge and the University of Sheffield as he gradually climbed the academic ladder. He returned to Oxford in 1935 as professor of pathology.

Two aspects of Florey's scientific approach especially distinguished him from Fleming. He was not intellectually bound by Wright's concepts of infectious disease, many of them theoretical; he was more inclined to do the experiment than to theorize about the probable outcome. He was also one of the first entrepreneurial researchers of our time, businesslike in the sense that he realized that the talents of various types of scientists would be needed to make important future breakthroughs in medicine. He, himself, was an accomplished physiologist-bacteriologist- pathologist, but he knew he would need the help of skilled biochemists in the work he envisioned at Oxford.

He turned to Cambridge for a likely candidate and finally accepted a young German Jewish refugee who had just completed a brilliant Ph.D. thesis there on the isolation of snake venom and the determination of its structure and action. This work of Ernst Boris Chain would prove a perfect preparation for the research that lay ahead at Oxford.

At thirty-seven years of age in 1935, Florey, the eminent professor of pathology at Oxford, had taken on many of the accoutrements of the establishment, at least outwardly. The animated young immigrant, ten years his junior, who physically resembled a youthful Einstein and was an accomplished pianist as well as a budding scientist, no doubt reminded him of his own arrival on the British scene fourteen years earlier.

By mid-1940 Florey had expanded his staff with other key figures who were expert in either bacteriology or biochemistry and who would prove invaluable. With each added staff member, Florey's efforts at obtaining grants to support them and meet their laboratory requirements were redoubled. This scrambling for support, importuning at every possible fount of potential research funds, was to plague Florey for much of his career.

The Oxford group concentrated on reexamining and analyzing the effects of various substances that had been reported to have antibacterial activity. Chain and his collaborator L. A. Epstein even followed up on the lysozyme work of Fleming and in 1938–39 were able to determine that it was an enzyme, a polysaccharidase. In reviewing other work in the field, Chain came upon Fleming's original paper concerning penicillin and obtained Florey's approval to reexplore this line of research. Within a year or two they had accumulated enough penicillin to attempt the animal experiments omitted by Fleming more than a decade earlier. MacFarlane, Florey's biographer, draws a vivid parallel between two events occurring on the morning of Saturday, May 25, 1940. While Britain's armed forces were making one of their historic military retreats at Dunkirk, Florey and his team began what was to prove one of her major historic medical advances. Eight mice were infected with equal lethal doses of streptococci; four later received penicillin. The four controls all died, whereas the treated mice survived. Larger groups of mice were subsequently studied, with similar success. The problem that now faced the researchers was to produce enough penicillin to conduct similar studies in the human being, three thousand times the size of a mouse.

Not only were methods needed to produce more penicillin, but it was also necessary to derive extracts of greater strength and purity. The seemingly potent material that they had used on the mice in 1940 was later shown to have a strength of only five units per milligram, whereas purified penicillin obtained several years later would have a strength of eighteen hundred units per milligram.

As the Oxford group confronted these problems, Florey decided to approach the pharmaceutical industry for help. With the war on, however, those best equipped to offer assistance were committed to the production of vaccines, antitoxins, and the study of blood substitutes and preservation. It was left to Florey and his colleagues to do the job themselves. A retelling of their superhuman efforts to achieve this feat would make a chapter in itself. Suffice it to say that they proved equal to the task. By February 1941, they were ready to apply their findings to patients.

A series of cases considered otherwise hopeless would constitute their first patients. The initial subject was a forty-three-year-old policeman with a severe combined streptococcal and staphylococcal infection involving the head, shoulder, and lungs. His condition had already proved refractory to surgical drainage and sulfa drugs. Penicillin treatment was followed by dramatic improvement, but after five days the supply ran out. Ten days later he relapsed and died. Five other seriously ill individuals then received penicillin, and in at least three a clear-cut cure was obtained. These promising results were published in the British medical journal *Lancet* in August 1941 and included many details of the laboratory techniques so painstakingly developed. In March of 1943 a much larger series, 187 cases in all, would be reported and conclusively demonstrate the effectiveness of penicillin in such infections.

Despite these successes, the aftermath of penicillin's introduction into clinical medicine would leave a bitter residue in the memories of all those at Oxford who had toiled so long and hard in that particular vineyard. To some extent Fleming, albeit unwittingly, must be held partly responsible for this.

The work at Oxford had proceeded without any input from Fleming. Indeed, all the while Chain had thought that Fleming had long since been dead. Fleming, for his part, must have been as surprised and pleased as anyone at the success in 1941 and a year later was able to act upon it personally.

In August 1942 a close friend of Fleming had developed streptococcal meningitis. When conventional therapy failed and death seemed imminent, Fleming turned to Florey for help. The latter personally delivered his remaining supply of penicillin to Fleming and instructed him in the initial use of it. A dramatic cure was obtained, even more so since penicillin was administered into the spinal canal for the first time to enhance its effectiveness. This "miracle" at St. Mary's was reported in the London *Times,* and the following day a letter from Almroth Wright identified Fleming as the one on whose brow the laurel wreath should rest. The rest of the press took up the story, and Fleming became a national hero overnight. Soon Oxford became all but forgotten in the public consciousness.

The reasons for such maldistribution of credit were multiple. Certainly Fleming, although he enjoyed all the attention, never claimed credit for anything more than he did. Others at St. Mary's were obviously responsible for exploiting this publicity. Wright wished to enhance the reputation of his department and Charles Wilson (Lord Moran), dean of St. Mary's Hospital Medical School, utilized the publicity for further advancement of the institution to which he had devoted much of his efforts.

Florey was galled by the self-promoting policies of St. Mary's and the lack of recognition for himself and his own devoted colleagues at Oxford. He was, however, trapped by the academic mores of the day. Such self-aggrandisement was deemed inappropriate and unseemly by the authorities at the Royal Society and the Medical Research Council. They told Florey to rest secure in the knowledge that the scientific community would recognize precisely where the true credit lay and that the future would vindicate him and his team at Oxford. The anticipated appreciation of posterity was little comfort to those at Oxford, and the enforced silence on the subject troubled them all for the remainder of their days.

The public aftermath of penicillin's triumph also poisoned Florey's relations with Chain. Chain, cognizant of the cutthroat nature of the pharmaceutical industry on the Continent, urged Florey to take out patents to protect certain aspects of penicillin production. Again the doyens of the British medical establishment prevailed upon Florey to desist, and later the British would learn to regret this oversight by having to pay royalties to American drug companies using the very techniques that they in Oxford had developed. On a trip to the United States to promote penicillin research, Florey left Chain behind in favor of another associate. Finally the British government refused to provide Chain with the technical resources he considered essential for his continued progress. In 1948 he left Oxford for another post at the Instituto Superiore di Sanita in Rome.

When Fleming, Florey, and Chain were called to Sweden to share in the Nobel prize in medicine, the crosscurrents of all these events were strongly reflected between the lines of their lectures.[5]

Chain acknowledged the help of his Oxford colleagues by name and then launched into a lengthy technical biochemical dissertation that was unlikely to be understood by any but a few of those present. Fleming, in essence, repeated the well-known "penicillin story" as it applied to him alone, emphasizing the important elements of lysozyme and the wartime study of antiseptics along the way.

Florey's presentation was the most curious. Using the excuse that he had recently lectured elsewhere on penicillin (as if this could have any possible bearing on so important an address as that of the Nobel ceremonies!), he then delivered a detailed lecture focusing first on all that went before the penicillin work at St. Mary's and Oxford and then on all that the future might bring. (Selman Waksman had recently introduced streptomycin, which would revolutionize the treatment of tuberculosis.) In the light of what we have come to know about the controversy regarding the history of penicillin, on reading this address today it seems as if, in emphasizing the distant past, Florey was indicating to us that Fleming's "discovery" of penicillin was just another in a long line of observations about the inhibition of one microorganism by another. Fleming, in all fairness to him, had freely acknowledged this, but the rest of the world seemed to have forgotten.*

While Chain and Florey tipped their hats to their coworkers the myth of Fleming's professional isolation—that is, his lack of biochemical assistance—was propagated by his own silence in this regard, although he acknowledged two others besides LaTouche in a forgotten footnote to his classic paper of 1929.

Also at St. Mary's were Drs. Frederick Ridley and Stuart Craddock. Although not formally trained in biochemistry, they had enough biochemical background and skill to determine some important aspects of penicillin's properties and means of extracting it. Craddock even went so far as volunteering as an experimental subject when he allowed Fleming to treat his chronic sinus infection with penicillin. This, however, as with much of the early tentative work with penicillin, was unsuccessful and did nothing to alter Flemings basically jaded view about its usefulness in deep-seated bacterial infection. Their work was forgotten and, at later dates, repeated by other workers unaware of these earlier findings.

Recalling Sir Isaac Newton's comment about "the shoulders

---

*Two others, it turns out, John Burdon-Sanderson, another St. Mary's man, in 1871 and Lord Lister himself in 1882, were the first to note the potentially beneficial effects of *Penicillium* mold. D. Zuck, "Who discovered penicillin? *World Medicine* (March 23, 1977): 60–65.

of giants," one must acknowledge that Fleming, Florey, and Chain were all gigantic. What the penicillin story ultimately demonstrates, however, is that lesser contributions as well as the elements of chance and luck are also important. It is the proper conjunction of *all* these elements that make up the essential matrix of scientific progress.

Turning Bad Luck into Good

The Alchemy of Willem Kolff, the First Successful Artificial Kidney and the Artificial Heart

It is Kampen, Holland, during the Nazi occupation. The medical officer from the local Wehrmacht garrison looks critically at the strange contraption before him and then addresses the tall, gangling Dutch physician beside it.[1]

"Ja. Das ist der Apparat den ich es aus der Literature Kenne." (Yes. This is the apparatus as I recognize it from the literature.)

He was bluffing, of course. Willem "Pim" Kolff, then in his thirties, had not yet published his findings concerning his new invention. When he did, however, it would completely revolutionize the treatment of acute and chronic renal failure and save or significantly prolong the lives of hundreds of thousands of patients over the next four decades.

Those who have devoted their lives to the study of the kidney have demonstrated that it is a remarkable and surprisingly versatile organ. It ensures that our blood volume neither expands excessively to overload us with fluid nor contracts to perilously low levels of dehydration with resultant underperfusion of our tissues and risk of developing shock. It keeps the hydrogen ion concentration optimal so that our body fluids become neither too acid nor too alkaline. It maintains the proper electrolyte mix for proper functioning of our cells and enzyme systems. It exerts an important effect on maintaining normal blood pressure. It helps to regulate red blood cell production. Finally, through its effects on clacium and phosphate excretion and retention, it is responsible for proper maintenance of the skeletal system, the scaffolding upon which depends all the rest of our body parts.

In short, the kidneys are vital in maintaining what the great French physiologist Claude Bernard more than a hundred years ago termed the "milieu interieur," which, if not properly maintained, could spell disaster for the organism.

So much for the experts. For the rest of us, less intimately acquainted with the complex mysteries of all those glomeruli and tubules that make up the kidney substance, it is simply an organ—or, rather, pair of organs—whose primary and most obvious function is the elimination of liquid waste. It is in this respect that malfunction of the kidneys has, for centuries, preoccupied physicians attending their patients with kidney failure. The uremic patient was a familiar if frustrating medical entity long before any of the more subtle functions of the kidney had been uncovered by renal physiologists.

Since the beginning of this century, students of kidney function had been aware that if they were to try substituting some external apparatus for the kidney's excretory function, they had to meet several important requirements. Among them was the need for a method to remove and return enough blood from the uremic subject so that adequate amounts of waste products could be eliminated over a reasonable period of time. Also required was a means of preventing blood from clotting while in transit through such an apparatus. Finally, it was necessary to find a membrane across which waste products would pass from the blood and into the device to result in the ultimate fall in their concentrations to normal levels within the patient.[2]

The membrane component requirement seems to have already been met, at least in part, in the nineteenth century. In 1854 a Scottish chemist, Thomas Graham, had reported in his paper, "On Osmotic Force," that, using a membrane fashioned from an ox bladder, he could effect the passage of solutes at high concentration in solution on one side of this semipermeable membrane across it to a solution with a lesser concentration of the same molecules. He termed this process "dialysis."

Before his death in 1901, Adolf Fick, a German scientist, made another important contribution to the membrane component of the prospective artificial kidney. He found that the syrupy liquid collodion, when dry, formed a porous membrane. This substance became the basic material for many experiments with dialysis thereafter.

The first complete apparatus developed for treatment of renal failure was developed in the laboratories of John Jacob Abel, a pharmacologist at Johns Hopkins University. There, in 1913, with his associates Leonard G. Rountree and B. B. Turner, he performed the first successful renal dialyses in dogs rendered uremic. Here for the first time the apparatus was given the name "artificial kidney."[3]

They utilized a collodion type of membrane, celloidin, formed into multiple tubes through which blood could flow. All this was mounted within a glass cylinder containing dialysis fluid to which the excretory products could pass from the blood. Heparin had not yet been discovered, so to keep the blood from clotting within the tubing they used as an anticoagulant, hirudin, extracted from the macerated heads of leeches, consuming literally thousands of these in their experiments.

The work of Abel and his coworkers was abruptly halted with the onset of World War I. Contact with Hungary, their source of leeches, was cut off and they were apparently either unaware of other sources or disinclined to use them. They had nonetheless demonstrated that an artificial kidney could work in experimental uremia and suggested its possible utility in certain cases of human kidney failure.

Although the First World War discouraged further studies of experimental uremia in Baltimore, it did serve to stimulate others, primarily in Germany, to pursue their own attempts at alleviating clinical uremia in humans. Dr. Heinrich Necheles of Hamburg was a medical student when drafted into the German army. When serving in a field hospital on the Western Front, he was horrified at the number of deaths from uremic coma in soldiers brought in from the battles.

"I thought, 'How could I prolong the lives of these lovely youngsters?' and that's how the thought of an artificial kidney grew within me."[4]

What made the need for treatment of such cases even more urgent was the growing realization that these battle wound cases represented cases of acute renal failure which would be followed by complete recovery if the patient's renal function could be artificially supported over the period of days or weeks it might take, depending upon the conditions leading to the shutdown. In crush injuries relating to war wounds, or other trauma with loss of blood, or in severe burn injuries with loss of blood volume leading to critical kidney underperfusion, acute reversible renal failure might ensue. It also became known that cases involving certain drugs, the early sulfa preparations and the antiseptic bichloride of mercury that was frequently used in suicide attempts, might also represent acute renal failure and thus be eminently suitable for such treatment.

Necheles, who, like Abel, also confined his work to the animal laboratory, used sheep peritoneum (lining of the abdominal cavity) as a dialyzing membrane. His major contribution to the development of an efficient artifical kidney was the recognition that a large surface area of membrane relative to blood would be necessary. This he accomplished by sandwiching multiple layers of peritoneum mounted on sheets of chicken wire screening arranged in series.

The first successful human hemodialyis (i.e. the removal of waste products from blood by dialysis) would be performed by another German, Dr. Georg Haas of the University Clinic at Giesen.[5] Haas is recalled as a somewhat unfulfilled figure because the value of his contributions was so poorly appreciated by the medical establishment at the time. He, too, was stimulated to study the possibility of human hemodialysis by the types of casualties he was called upon to treat during the First World War.

Apparently, during all of his initial efforts, he was totally unaware of the work of Abel and his associates owing to the breakdown in scientific communication as a result of the Great War. However, his own scientific background prior to the war made him uniquely qualified to undertake such studies on his own. He had devised dialysis techniques, for example, in his study of amino acid metabolism in dogs while in Strasbourg.

Despite all this, Haas's wartime efforts came to nought. Among other problems, he could not prepare suitable dialyzing membranes, and the crude hirudin that was available was difficult to work with and often toxic. His hemodialysis project was abandoned in the middle of the war when he was sent to the Eastern Front to help combat an outbreak of typhus in Romania.

In the postwar years Haas's interest was rekindled by the published researches of Necheles and his awareness that celloidin might serve as a suitable dialyzing membrane. He also then learned of the work of Abel and his group in the United States and began a correspondence with the Johns Hopkins pharmacologist. He resumed his dog work, training himself in the construction of an artificial kidney very similar in design to that of Abel. A more purified, less toxic form of hirudin also became available for these new efforts.

By the autumn of 1924 Haas was ready to attempt the first human hemodialysis and, with the assistance of a surgical colleague, performed without complications a fifteen-minute dialysis in a patient with terminal uremia. In February of 1925 a second dialysis was performed by Haas, this time for thirty-five minutes, using a continuous circulation technique—blood being drawn and returned to the patient almost simultaneously. Except for a mild febrile reaction, again the procedure was well tolerated.

Further attempts at dialysis were made by Haas over the next four years with promising but inconclusive results about its practicality for routine clinical use.

Haas's caution in his predictions was partially based on the continuing problems he encountered with obtaining adequate blood flow through his devices, although he attempted to achieve this by designing a mechanical pumping system to meet this requirement. A greater problem was the need for hirudin during the early stages of this research. The latter problem was solved with the discovery of heparin in 1916 (again it was at Johns Hopkins), although the product did not become commercially available for many years thereafter. Haas, after many trials and failures, finally succeeded in producing his own heparin for his dialysis studies.

By 1928 Haas, although only forty-two and still vigorous, gave up his work on the artificial kidney. One wonders why. By this time, he had overcome many of the technical problems in human hemodialysis that had previously beset him. He had pretty well solved the anticoagulation problem with the availability of heparin; he had devised a pump to facilitate transport of blood from the back to the patient. He had achieved some unquestionable successes—and then he stopped.

It is difficult to fathom why he did not go on. A shy and reticent man, he never expounded on this in his writings. A surviving nephew, when contacted, was mute on the subject. It has been suggested that politics involving other investigators, perhaps Necheles among them, blocked acceptance of his methods.[6] Undoubtedly, many conventional practitioners thought that hemodialyis was too extreme a means of controlling uremia and chose to continue the traditional methods of bloodletting, forced sweating, and dietary restriction of protein to ward off the terminal stage.

At this time in his life, Haas had also begun to rise in stature at the Giessen clinic, where he assumed administrative duties as head of the medical section. As so often happens in such instances, the research tends to get squeezed out. Perhaps he had simply reached a point at which, as an innovator, he was *ausgespielt* ("played out"). He had given the problem his best shot; it was now for others to carry on. Whatever the explanation, except for subsequent gentle reminders about his place in the history of dialysis when others happened to forget it, George Haas withdrew from active research.

The years between the wars were strangely uneventful for progress in artificial kidney research. This hiatus, during which one might possibly have expected rational and systematic study of the problem, contained only a few nuggets of worthwhile research. For example, newly purified heparin became available. There was also a significant finding that came from a rather unusual source—the sausage-making industry.

Meat-packing firms had begun to mass produce cellophane as casing for their sausage products. In 1937, Dr. William Thalheimer, a former student of Abel, determined that this readily available and cheap material could also serve as an excellent dialyzing membrane. In future work on the artificial kidney, it became an essential ingredient for success.

It took another world war to push ahead the development of the artificial kidney; another world war and Willem Kolff.

The son of a physician who had been in charge of a tuberculosis sanitorium, Kolff, as a boy, had no desire to follow in his father's footsteps. The problems involved with attempting to treat incurable tuberculosis were often too much for father Kolff, and his son recalls seeing him in tears, at times, so frustrating and saddening were these experiences. Nevertheless, Kolff's mind changed as he approached manhood and he graduated as a physician from the University of Leiden in 1938 and took a teaching post at the University of Groningen.

There he came under the influence of two men. Professor R. Brinkman was a biochemist who introduced him to the dialyzing properties of cellophane with which Kolff conducted his first crude experiments, filling sausage casing with blood and measuring the removal of urea from the blood after he agitated the "blood sausage" in a bath of physiological salt solution. Pollak Daniels was the head of the Department of Medicine. From him, Kolff received encouragement to proceed in exploring new ideas no matter how foolish or impractical the "experts" around might deem them.

Early in his clinical work at Groningen, Kolff became acutely sensitized to the plight of patients, especially young ones, with renal failure. At the time, no one was doing anything about it, and Kolff resolved to have a try. The work in Groningen, however, was abruptly interrupted by the German invasion in 1940.

On the day of the assault Kolff and his wife were in the Hague planning to attend the funeral of her grandfather. As the Luftwaffe appeared overhead delivering bombs as well as pamphlets calling for surrender, Kolff rushed to the main hospital to see if he could be of assistance. Anticipating the arrival of wounded, he inquired if any blood-banking provisions had been made. There had been no such planning. His offer to set up a blood bank was accepted, and, in a truck with a soldier beside him to protect against snipers, he rushed about the city picking up bottles, tubing, needles, and so on. The result was the first blood bank of its kind in Europe, and Kolff proudly points out that it is still in existence.

With the ensuing Nazi takeover of the country, Kolff's position at Groningen became untenable for him. Pollak and his wife, both Jews, took their own lives in anticipation of what they could expect at the hands of the invaders. The Germans then rejected the candidate presented by the Groningen faculty to succeed Pollak and named their own man to fill the vacancy, a Dutch Nazi.

Kolff resolved that he would never serve under such a man and left before the new department head could assume his office. Kolff recalled that on his way back to Groningen from the Hague, he had stopped at the ancient town of Kampen on the Ijsel River. He had struck up a conversation with the mayor there and learned that the local ninety-bed hospital was seeking a full-time internist. At this point being jobless, Kolff indicated that he was available.

Although Kolff was the youngest candidate for the position and the most demanding in terms of what he required in updating of equipment and other supplies, it was he who was selected for the post, suffering only a short "lay-off" in the time between his departure from Groningen and the assumption of his new duties.

While at Groningen, Kolff had had a prototype of his artificial kidney constructed for him by a local manufacturer, but it was not until he arrived in Kampen that he began to make real progress.

By this time, heparin was available for the prevention of blood clotting, and he had a suitable membrane in the form of his sausage casings. His major personal contribution in devising a new design for the artificial kidney lay in a method of ensuring adequate rates of delivery of blood to and from the apparatus. The presence in Kampen of a Mr. H. Berk and supplies from his enamel factory, the town's main industry, enabled the budding nephrologist to achieve this success. The solution is best described in Kolff's own words:

> After my initial experience with sausage casings in Groningen, simple arithmetic dictated that I would have to use tubing at least ten or twenty meters long with one half to a liter of blood in order to dialyze a patient adequately. This was finally accomplished by wrapping twenty meters of cellophane tubing around a horizontally placed drum, which in turn was placed in a trough containing dialysis solution. Any blood within the tubing sinks by gravity to the lowest point in the drum, and as the drum is rotated with its lower half in dialysate, the blood is constantly coming in contact with the solution through the tubing, of course. Now, the blood has to get into one end of the cellophane tubing wrapped around the drum and then out the other end. This was best done by leading it through the hollow axle of the drum. We first tried rubber rotating couplings for connecting the tubes to and from the patient to the rotating drum but had some trouble with them. They kept getting twisted as the drum rotated. I then went to see the local Ford dealer and took over the idea that Henry Ford had used in constructing the seal of the water pump of his engine. I copied it, having only to drill a hole in it for my purposes. The first artificial kidneys had drums made of aluminum around which the cellophane tubing was wrapped. When aluminum could no longer be obtained due to wartime shortages, we used wooden lathes. They worked fine, except that often the wood was not aged properly and warped.

This was not the last time that Kolff would go beyond his immediate medical circles to seek assistance. He has never hesitated to use nonmedical people like Berk when they are the ones who can provide the solution to a pressing problem. ("I'll take a good technician over a mediocre doctor any day.") However, in addition to Berk, Kolff was fortunate in having at the Kampen hospital a small but devoted team of doctors and nurses to assist him.

An incurable and eclectic gadgeteer, he would later adapt orange juice cans and a commercial clothes washer to meet the requirements of future devices of his design. At Kampen, however, even the most simple supplies were in short supply. Kolff had the foresight to buy up large quantities of cellophane casings before coming to Kampen, but throughout his stay there he ran into constant shortages of such simple and basic items as rubber tubing and needles.

As if to add to all the difficulties he was having in maintaining his equipment in working order, the inital results with the Kolff artificial kidney could hardly have been considered encouraging to anyone, with the possible exception of Kolff himself. Between March 1943 and July 1944 treatment of fifteen patients resulted in only one survivor, and even that success could not really be attributed to treatment with the artificial kidney. It involved a young man who, following treatment with one of the early sulfa drugs, went into acute renal failure after the drug had crystallized and blocked off his ureters. It was really relief of the mechanical obstruction rather than treatment with dialysis that was the key to his recovery.

In later years, after his exasperating experiences of wrangling with various levels of the American medical bureaucracy, Kolff would reflect that if those early failures had occurred in his adopted country, given such a climate, he would never have been permitted to continue. In Holland, convinced that he was on the right track, he was able to push on.

The first real success took place in September 1945 with a sixty-seven-year-old woman, Sophia Schafstadt, who was brought to Kolff in uremic coma due to acute renal failure. She recovered consciousness, receiving eleven hours of dialysis in the process, and lived another seven years before succumbing to another illness. Ironically, Kolff the Dutch patriot and political liberal had had as his initial triumph a Nazi sympathizer who was believed to have betrayed many of her countrymen to the Germans.

Kolff remains philosophical about this. "If a patient needs help to save his life you give that help and don't ask whether he is a National Socialist [Nazi] or anything else."

Following the experience with Schafstadt, further successes were obtained, but Kolff's work on the artificial kidney was interrupted by the realities of war. The Germans, when finally about to retreat from the Netherlands, decided to transport a large part of the Dutch male population to Germany to work on fortifications. Indiscriminately, they rounded up all the males in Rotterdam, loaded them on large coal barges, eight hundred prisoners to each, and towed them across the Zuider Zee to Kampen. From this point, they would be transported by train to Germany.

Among the prisoners were the deaf and blind, paralytics, mental defectives, diabetics who had no insulin, all tossed headlong into this mass evacuation. One morning, with over eight thousand of these prisoners on barges docked at Kampen, a local doctor approached Kolff to help him save those who would most certainly perish otherwise. Kolff appraised the situation and then requested permission from the German commander to take the sick off the barges and care for them.

"Who will be responsible? All these people are terrorists," the officer replied. Kolff said that he, personally, would take responsibility.

"Very well," said the officer, "but if they run away, you will be shot."

Knowing of the Germans' passion for record keeping, Kolff and his assistants planned to give them just what they wanted. With the help of some of the prisoners, businessmen and accountants knowledgeable about such things, they set up an elaborate card-file system designed to hide the fact that, in addition to pulling the sick and disabled off the barges, they were helping resistance fighters, Jews, and others escape their captors.

Kolff recalls, "I wasn't very fat when I started, but during that last winter I lost another twenty pounds!"

Despite the hardships of the war and the shortage of materials, by the end of the war Kolff and his team had a number of successful studies under their collective belt and had published these results in Swiss, French, and Scandinavian medical journals. They had also been able to construct additional units, of which they sent samples to Great Britain, Canada, and providentially, Mt. Sinai Hospital in New York.

It was the final offer that gained Kolff his entrée to the United States, and this was through the intercession of another remarkable Dutchman, Dr. Isadore Snapper.[7]

Snapper (1889–1973) had been something of a wunderkind in prewar Holland, having been appointed full professor of medicine at the University of Amsterdam at the tender age of thirty, an accomplishment as rare then as it would be today. His expertise as an internist spanned many fields within it both in physiological chemistry and at the bedside. Like Kolff, he had been displaced by the war, but Snapper's odyssey was much more worthy of the name.

In 1938, possibly foreseeing the Nazi domination of Europe and, as a Jew, cognizant of exactly what that might mean to him, Snapper left Holland for the Peking Union Medical College in China. Eventually, he fell into the hands of the Japanese but regained his freedom and came to the United States after being exchanged for a Japanese general who had been held by the Dutch. For a short time he served as a consultant to the office of the Surgeon General before taking up a position at Mt. Sinai, where he remained between 1944 and 1952.

In 1947, Kolff, who had not known Snapper before, despite their common heritage, wrote to the older man, sending reprints and offering, along with the donation of an artificial kidney, a personal demonstration on how to use it. Snapper arranged an invitation which led to the first successful human dialysis in the United States. The success of the Mt. Sinai visit led Snapper to arrange for Kolff to visit a number of other teaching hospitals. Among these was Harvard's Peter Bent Brigham Hospital from which would later emanate an improved model of Kolff's kidney, designed with his assistance.

In 1949 Kolff returned to the United States actively seeking a position. Unlike the many American servicemen-physicians who were returning to complete their hospital training and who could depend on the G.I. Bill of Rights for economic support, the impecunious Kolff had no external means of support but did have a wife and four children with a fifth soon to be on the way. He had no choice but to seek a post that would enable him to support them, and such positions were not readily available.

Why was it so important for him to leave Holland at all? For one thing, like many other Europeans, Kolff suspected that the Russians might soon be overrunning all of Europe. Holland, with the loss of its colonies, was becoming more crowded and had an uncertain future. But what made it most imperative in Kolff's mind to make such a move had nothing to do with such general considerations or even the future of his artificial kidney. He knew that at a small, community ninety-bed hospital such as that in Kampen, he could never proceed with his next project, a heart-lung machine that would allow for open-heart surgery. For this, he would need a large institution with a talented multidisciplinary staff of medical specialists and surgeons who could bring it off.

All this he thought would come to pass when he was offered and accepted a position at the presitigious Cleveland Clinic in 1950. He had previously corresponded with their most preeminent researcher, Dr. Irvine H. Page, who had concentrated his efforts on mechanisms of hypertension and had been codiscoverer of the pressor substance angiotensin. Kolff had suggested that with Page's expertise in hypertension and his own skill in dialysis, they would make a powerful team.

Soon after he arrived in Cleveland, however, he found to his dismay that what Page had in mind was something quite different. He wanted Kolff simply to assist him in his own areas of research, and as for dialysis, "he became very unfriendly." The fate of the heart-lung machine was even worse. At that time, the surgeons at the Cleveland Clinic, as well as elsewhere, were concentrating on the recently introduced closed mitral commissurotomy, which involved the surgeon blindly putting a finger through the left atrium and opening up a narrowed rheumatic mitral valve. The shortcomings and complications of such a blind procedure were yet to be realized, and the surgeons were not receptive at the time to any complicated newfangled apparatus such as Kolff had in mind. Kolff simply had to put his heart-lung machine in storage and, like American surgeon John Gibbon, who had been working on a similar device for bypassing the heart interoperatively since 1935, had to wait for the rest of the medical world to catch up in its thinking.

In the ensuing years, many advances were made in improving the design of subsequent artificial kidneys, many of them attributable to Kolff himself. Peritoneal dialysis, although not having originated with Kolff and his group in Kampen, had been tested there intensively, especially by Kolff's associate Dr. Piet Kop who published the first important monograph on this technique. In contrast to hemodialyis, where blood is drawn through the artificial kidney to clear it of its wastes, in peritoneal dialysis several liters of dialysis fluid are introduced through the abdominal wall into the abdominal cavity of the patient. The lining of the abdominal cavity, the peritoneum, serves as the dialyzing membrane, and the blood flowing through the structures therein is able to unload urea and other substances to the dialysate, which is later removed.

Paramount in the growing understanding of the role of dialysis in the treatment of uremia was the recognition by investigators of the distinction between acute and chronic renal failure. Real success at first could only be achieved with the first since, after the crisis period had passed, patients could look forward to complete recovery and a normal lifespan. With chronic renal failure, or end-stage renal disease as it is also called, life could be prolonged only by repeating dialysis twice or thrice weekly over a period of months or years. The major problem with this treatment was the need for repeated access to blood vessels from which blood could be drawn and then returned to the patient.

This obstacle was partly solved by Drs. Belding Scribner and Wayne Quinton of the University of Washington medical school in Seattle. What they did was construct an external Teflon shunt between an artery and vein in the forearm to provide convenient access for repeated dialyses. Although a great improvement on the prior state of affairs, the Scribner shunt was subject to infection, dislodgement, and other problems inherent to such an externally placed construction. In 1966, this shunt was superseded by an innovation of Dr. James Cimino at New York University's Bellevue Hospital. He constructed a connection between a forearm vein and artery—an artificial arteriovenous fistula—that provided an internal conduit that could repeatedly be used as the shunt developed into a large thick-walled tube under the skin into which needles leading to the artificial kidney could be repeatedly introduced.

Perhaps one of the most important developments in the story of the artificial kidney, in the United States at least, was more of a political than a scientific event. In the 1960s, as hemodialysis began to prove itself as an effective long-term procedure, the major problem became how to finance it. Throughout this time and into the early 1970s, as more and more patients clamored to be admitted to such programs which had to be supported by other than patient-derived funds, what came to be recognized as life-or-death committees came into being at dialysis centers throughout the United States. Given their limited resources, it became the duty of such panels to determine which patients most merited admission to their limited chronic dialysis programs. Kidney specialists and others responsible for making such agonizing decisions were relieved of this burden in 1972, when the United States Congress passed legislation as part of the Medicare Act to ensure support for treatment of all future patients clinically found suitable for such care.

Meanwhile, through many of these developments, after five years in the shadow of Page, Kolff, step by step found it possible to assert himself at the clinic, resume his work on the artificial kidney, and, with the surgeons' increasing awareness of the shortcomings of the closed mitral commissurotomy procedure, pull his heart-lung bypass equipment out of the closet and resume work on this new, even more challenging problem. Much of this he was able to accomplish by wearing two hats within the Cleveland Clinic, with appointments in both the Department of Surgery and the Department of Research. When some new idea or program was blocked in one department, he usually found it possible to bring it to fruition in the other. All this came to an end in 1967, when he was informed that he would have to confine his activities thereafter to only one department. The same night Kolff began looking for a new job.

Learning that the University of Utah in Salt Lake City had one of the best regional medical programs in the country, he turned westward. When assured of adequate cooperation from the Department of Surgery and facilitation of his grant requests with a minimum of interference from the bureaucracy, Kolff decided that this was the place where he could really move ahead with his artificial organ program. He accepted a position at the University of Utah as a professor of surgery at the medical school, heading its Division of Artificial Organs. True to form, Kolff also arranged to get an appointment to the College of Engineering as research professor and head of the Institute for Biomedical Engineering.

Although Kolff's work on the artificial kidney has been the main basis for his public recognition, his contributions to other types of artificial organ development have also been recognized as seminal by those more intimately involved in such matters. Even during the war, in Holland he had begun work on the heart-lung machine, which would permit open-heart surgery. Eventually he was able to continue this work in Cleveland with the cooperation of such cardiac surgeons as Dr. Donald B. Effler. While at Cleveland, Kolff and his colleagues also worked on the aortic balloon device for the treatment of cardiogenic shock states, a procedure later popularized by surgeon Adrian Kantrowitz and others.

In Utah he was able to branch out into a number of fields. In the cardiovascular area, Kolff's group came up with a left-ventricular assist device. Substantial progress was made with development of and miniaturization for a practical artificial ear. By stimulation of the surface of the brain with electrodes, even artificial sight came within their purview, although a

roomful of instrumentation was still necessary for its operation when this work was temporarily halted a few years ago.
The most dramatic of all these new developments, of course,
was the artificial heart, upon which Kolff and Dr. Tetsuzo
Akutsu had already performed work in Cleveland and demonstrated its feasibility in dogs back in 1957.

Although many cardiac patients could be helped by surgery
for congenital defects, valvular disease, or coronary heart disease by open-heart procedures devised during the 1960s and
1970s, there was still a significant number whose hearts were
so damaged that only complete replacement of the organ
could offer any hope for survival.

Complete heart transplantation from appropriate donors
was one option, but the supply was limited and only relatively
few patients could therefore benefit. The other option was the
artificial heart, and it was toward this end that the efforts of
Kolff and his associates became increasingly directed.

In Utah Kolff continued the work in experimental animals,
determined one day to apply it to humans. As the work progressed, Kolff was told of a young American medical student
who was disinclined to return to Bologna to continue studies
there because of political unrest in the country. The young
man had an engineering background and some interesting
ideas. Kolff hired Robert Jarvik, who finally designed the artificial heart model that would be placed in the first human recipient.

At the University of Utah another medical student came to
Kolff's attention, one who went on to Duke to complete a thoracic surgery residency. When he returned to Utah, William
DeVries was well equipped to fulfill the surgical demands of
the team.

In December of 1982, a retired dentist, sixty-one-year-old
Barney Clark, was near death from heart failure that had become refractory to all conventional medical therapy. He became the first recipient of the Jarvik heart and survived for
112 days before succumbing to multiple complications involving the kidneys, lungs, and infection. Several other patients
succeeded him, but problems with infection and the formation

of blood clots that formed within the device and then broke off, embolizing to vital organs such as the brain, proved, for the present, insurmountable. No active program for permanent insertion of an artificial heart is now in operation, although such devices are proving helpful in bridging the time it takes to obtain human donor hearts for some moribund cardiac patients.

In the aftermath of these first attempts with the artificial heart, the paths of these three have separated. Jarvik and DeVries have left Utah. Not generally appreciated is the contribution that Kolff's nurturing of their talents made to their subsequent careers and the future of the artificial heart program.

About this aspect of his career and, indeed, all of his former work and its future application, Kolff remains pragmatically clear-eyed. Despite all of the work that he has put into the artificial kidney, he makes no bones about his belief that it has no place in the future treatment of end-stage renal disease. The success of cyclosporine and its possible successors as well as better tissue typing to prevent rejection has made kidney transplantation not only desirable but practical. In the best of all possible future worlds, he sees transplantation replacing chronic dialysis. For the future of the artificial heart, he has a different scenario. While we all have two kidneys and can live with one; while we can frequently use cadaver kidneys in transplant work; we have only one heart each, and the supply that can be harvested from auto accident victims and similar patients with brain death but sturdy hearts will never meet the need for the thirty to fifty thousand or more hearts each year in the United States alone. The artificial heart is the only answer.

Thus far the externally powered artificial heart has run into problems, but about this and future developments Kolff remains optimistic. And with good reason, based on his past experiences. ("Calamities and disasters have turned out to my advantage in the long run.")

Under the worst of wartime conditions, he set up the first blood bank of its kind in Europe, one that continues to flourish. Under no less adverse conditions, he devised the first practical artificial kidney for hemodialysis. Despite his great hopes for new opportunities at the Cleveland Clinic, he met repeated opposition, but still managed to improve his design of the artificial kidney and advance his work on the heart-lung bypass machine.

Even in Utah, the most favorable of all his bases of operation, it has been far from a smooth sail. On one occasion he found that a large number of the sheep he had been using for development of the artificial heart had been stolen. In that year they had sufficient research funds. In the following year, when research support faltered, the insurance money from the stolen sheep enabled the program to survive. Later on, in 1973, his laboratory was consumed in flames. They thought it irreplaceable. The one that they built by renovating the outdated premises of a local hospital resulted in one of the most advanced experimental laboratories for artificial organs in the world.

Kolff has had some federal support for grants, but never enough and always with ample doses of aggravation thrown in. He has seen his own ideas and those of his group rejected by granting agencies, that subsequently funded such research at other laboratories. The National Institute of Health was dead set against the Utah team implanting an artifical heart, but the Secretary of Health came to the rescue by placing this decision in the hands of the Food and Drug Administration, which looked upon this experimental trial more favorably.

Dr. Kolff has good reason to remain optimistic. After all, who else has demonstrated so many times and in so many different places that under the worst of conditions bad luck can indeed be turned into good?

Say It Isn't "No"

The Power of Positive Thinking in the Publication of Medical Research

Harvard's C. Sydney Burwell is credited with a remark to the effect that half of what we teach our medical students will, in time, be shown to be wrong but that, unfortunately, we do not know which half. To my knowledge, no one has ever seriously challenged this. If the statement is indeed true, logic would dictate that much of current medical research would be devoted to correcting the fallacies of the past and that our journals would be full of the re-search to set us straight.

On the contrary, on perusing the medical literature, I have often been struck by the dominance of those investigators with positive findings, with the nay sayers in a distinct minority. On a personal level, it has always been those studies of mine that have challenged some previously reported data or beliefs that have had the most trouble getting published. Particularly galling about such rejections was the fact that these investigations were frequently the most difficult, tedious, and meticulously performed. It seemed, at times, that the only way to get ahead was to be a perpetual yes man.

In younger days I used to brood about this. As I grew older, I began to philosophize about it. What finally nudged these thoughts into print was the passing of Dr. Julius Comroe. Aside from his many academic interests and contributions at both the University of Pennsylvania and the Cardiovascular Research Institute at the University of California in San Francisco, he was vitally interested in exactly how and why research is pursued. Certain of his writings such as his book, *Retrospectroscope*, and essay *Ben Franklin and Open Heart Surgery* should be required reading for anyone who even pretends to be interested in doing research.[1]

I recall an address on such matters that Dr. Comroe delivered to a large audience of clinical researchers. Tongue-in-cheek, he confessed that in his own career he had once committed a grievous error. He had attempted to repeat a previously successful experiment—and failed. Before committing myself to a grievous error in print, I felt obliged to attempt some verification of my impressions about the power of positive research and the difficulties in gaining an audience for negative results. There were previous studies I knew about on the types of medical research performed, the changing productivity of investigators, the ethics of human research, and even the number of authors on papers published over the years, but none about negative research. The *Index Medicus* does not even include the term and a MEDLARS search for it under various guises proved fruitless.

An examination of this question was certainly in order, then, and what better place to start than an excellent general medical journal such as *The New England Journal of Medcine?* For the calendar year 1984 I reviewed all the original articles and classified them according to the conclusions reached as having positive findings, negative results, or neither (neutral studies on the basis of inconclusive or mixed results). Excluded were articles on less than five patients, those of a nature inapplicable to the categorization planned, and those I simply could not understand. Since the purpose of this exercise was merely to confirm or deny a personal impression and not convince any cadre of statisticians that might be lying in wait for me at some editorial office, no formal evaluations of statistical significance were attempted. I refused to be undone by a p value.

Of the 208 articles I reviewed, 168 were positive in their

conclusions, 20 negative, and 20 neutral (80 percent, 10 percent, and 10 percent, respectively). Did this low number of negative studies, given the Burwell dictum, indicate anything idiosyncratic about the *New England Journal* in its selection of papers to be published? To check on this, the first hundred papers for 1984 in a specialty journal, the *Annals of Internal Medicine*, per unit were similarly reviewed: 89 percent positive, 1 percent negative and 10 percent neutral. The results from a similar analysis in the *Annals of Surgery:* 91 percent positive, 3 percent negative, and 6 percent neutral. If anything, the *New England Journal* was even *less* Panglossian in its view of medical research than the others.

It occurred to me that perhaps there might be more room for the admission of doubt among the abstracts presented at a medical meeting. After all, none of these presentations would automatically become part of the medical literature. Of one hundred presented papers randomly selected for review from the 1984 annual meeting of the American Federation for Clinical Research, 95 percent turned out to be positive, 2 percent negative, and 3 percent neutral.* One must conclude that it pays to be positive.

As for the reverse, the Bad News Bearers of medical research have never fared as well. This is something of a mystery, especially when one recalls how often we have been victimized by our own collective overenthusiasm and gullibility. The effects of such lapses in good judgment can be disastrous in terms of impeding scientific progress.

The flub of the century in this regard probably belongs to Professor Johannes Fibiger, the Danish pathologist who first found worms in the stomach cancers of rats in 1907 and made a connection. By the time 1913 rolled around, he had reported his work on the experimental induction of spiroptera

---

*Of interest regarding this group of papers is research indicating that over a year's time following such meetings, fewer than half the abstracts submitted may actually result in permanent publications. L. Goldman and A. Loscalzo, "Fate of cardiology research originally published in abstract form," *New Engl. J Med* 303 (1980): 255.

carcinoma in rodents.[2] For this, "the greatest contribution to experimental medicine in our generation," (according to his introduction at the Nobel ceremonies), he was awarded the Nobel Prize in Medicine and Physiology in 1926.[3] This "immortal research" (ditto) was never duplicated. Meanwhile, Peyton Rous, who was really on to something in 1910 when, at the Rockefeller Institute, he demonstrated the transfer of chicken sarcomas with a cell-free filtrate, was virtually ignored for his contribution to understanding the association between viruses and cancer.[4] It was "once bitten twice shy" for the Nobel committees when it came to giving awards for cancer after Fibiger, and it was only in 1966, after over half a century and more than twenty nominations that Rous, then eighty-seven, finally received his just recognition in Stockholm.

Fibiger, whatever the error of his work, could not be faulted for lack of sincerity or honesty. He, at least, did not mean to mislead us. But there were mental aberrants who were just as successful in leading the scientific community astray. Cyril Burt, the English psychologist who dominated the field in the 1930s and 1940s, and whose work on separated identical twins was critical to the position of those who insisted on the primacy of inheritance in intelligence, manufactured not only twin pairs out of thin air but collaborators as well. John Darsee, a case study in psychopathic behavior if there ever was one, was a shooting star in the field of cardiology only a few years ago. In his ascendancy he dazzled his superiors both at Emory University and then Harvard Medical School with his brilliance and productivity. He cleverly mixed up valid work with his faked creations which may have provided him with something of a smokescreen. But why were they so successful for so long? There were certainly many critical minds in England as well as at Emory and Harvard while the papers were churned out. Although many factors can be implicated, the simple desire of all around them to glow in the reflection of all those lovely positive results must have been a major consideration, one gathers from reading the interviews of those concerned.

Still, whatever the source of the misinformation involved, it is a comfort to realize that sometime, somewhere there will be someone who will take a very close look. Fortunately there are those among us who have an almost unreasonable persistence in pursuing their hunches even when previous evidence is to the contrary. There are also those with a persnickety compulsion to prove to themselves that what others have found is really correct. It is they, the doubting heroes of this piece, who help redress the imbalance induced by both those in honest error and those who lie.

Perhaps it was this sort of attitude that prompted Tijo and Levan, thirty-three years after the number of human chromosomes had been established as forty-eight, to hold a recount and find, with newer techniques, that it was really forty-six.[5] This kind of thinking was surely instrumental in motivating Dr. George Cotzias and his associates at Brookhaven Laboratories to pursue their levodopa work in the treatment of Parkinsonism when others had reported lack of persistent improvement in patients and unacceptable side effects.[6] Alterations in dosage and administration regimens by the Brookhaven group solved both of these problems to the extent that such therapy became a mainstay in the treatment of this disease.

It took decades for the moment of truth to emerge but, thanks to Princeton's Leon Kamin, the forgeries of Burt, through his own statistical analyses, were uncovered.[7] Fraud can even have a brighter side after those hard to convince have exposed it. It was the failure of others at Sloan-Kettering and elsewhere to repeat William Summerlin's experiments with mouse skin transplantation that set the search for explanations in motion. Summerlin, unable to repeat his transplants successfully after his transfer from Minnesota to New York, was pressured by criticism into finally presenting his superior, Robert Good, with the now famous painted mice. But the aftermath of the scandal also provided good science. It was found that, in coming to New York, Summerlin had, unconsciously, altered the conditions of the experiment. When these were later rectified, success was once again obtained.

Such dramatic episodes underline the importance of reassessing the body of medical knowledge. What they do not tell us is how much of that body needs to be reassessed. There are holes that can easily be poked in the analysis undertaken here. For example, many of the articles printed are not really the results of experiments but simply descriptive or epidemiological information about certain diseases that should not fall into the category of grading imposed here. Another type of report, a new test for something, if it had failed in the originator's laboratory, would certainly have no place cluttering up the literature. So all of these reports would naturally be positive. What about all the ideas and pilot studies we personally perform and reject that never even reach the journal submission stage? Granting all this room for error, one can still point to figures that are impressive.

One final question might be asked. "Was Burwell really wrong in the first place?" Could it be that there is *not* that large amount of false information lying about awaiting correction? Could this then account for the paucity of negative reports in the literature? I sought a clue by taking another, closer look at those articles in the *New England Journal*.

I tried to determine which of them really attempted to reassess either a previous study or a current practice. Although it soon became apparent that a certain degree of subjectivity could not be avoided in such a selection, I plunged right in.

There were, among the 208 articles, thirty-seven that could be classified as a reexamination of previous research. Of these, eighteen confirmed the prior work, ten denied it, and nine were inconclusive. On the basis of this one might suspect that Burwell was very close to the mark if not right on it. One might even suspect that editors, at least some of them, are not all that prone to "accentuate the positive, eliminate the negative." But I would like to "keep the book open" on that one.

An Anemia Called "Pernicious"

In 1849, Dr. Thomas Addison of Guy's Hospital in London read a paper before the South London Medical Society. In it he remarked, "For a long period I had, from time to time, met with a remarkable form of general anemia occurring without any discernable cause whatsoever." Although he later became famous for the diseases resulting in destruction of the adrenal glands, disorders that still bear his name, he also described the clinical manifestations of this blood disease in an unforgettable way.

> It makes its approach in so slow and insidious a manner that the patient can hardly fix a date to his earliest feeling of that languour which is shortly to become so extreme. The countenance gets pale, the whites of the eyes become pearly, the general frame flabby . . . ; there is an increasing indisposition to exertion . . . ; the whole surface of the body presents a blanched, smooth and waxy appearance; the lips, gums and tongue seem bloodless; . . . the appetite fails; extreme languor and faintness supervene, breathlessness and palpitations being produced by the most trifling exertion or emotion, . . . The patient can no longer rise from his bed, the mind occasionally wanders, he falls into a prostrate and torpid state, and at length expires.

Although it would be left to others to emphasize the neurological findings and atrophy of the stomach which are part and parcel to the disease, Addison's bedside description of it, even at this late date, after generations of hematologists, bio-chemists, and molecular biologists have had their say, remains vivid and compelling. It was in 1872 that Professor Anton Biermer in Switzerland attached the modifier *perniciöser* ("per-nicious") to the disorder, and the name stuck. It would take another fifty years, however, until any effective treatment would be found and even longer before the real cause of it could be determined.

Pernicious anemia (PA) was not only mysterious, but far from uncommon and always deadly. It was most prevalent among those of English, Irish, and Scandinavian ancestry and would occur during what we would now consider the prime of life, between the ages of thirty and sixty-five. In the United States alone, by 1926, the year the first effective treatment would be discovered, it was established that approximately six thousand patients were dying annually from the disease, most of them within one to three years of its onset.

To understand better how this particular medical mystery was unravelled, it helps to know a few facts at the onset: some-thing about how red blood cells are formed; why they are not produced in adequate number in PA; and, in order to appre-ciate the reasons for the many false starts and blind alleys of the past, some idea of what doctors thought about anemias in earlier times.

The normal production of red blood cells (erythrocytes) is now well known to be dependent on a number of dietary fac-tors. Protein is required, as are minerals such as iron and cop-per and a number of vitamins: folic acid, B_6, B_2, and, of course, B_{12} (cyanocobalamin). The last of these, the lack of which leads to PA, is unique in that not only must it be in-cluded in our diet from a variety of animal sources, but two crucial steps are involved in order for our bodies to absorb it. First, the ingested B_{12} must be bound in the stomach to a pro-tein found in normal gastric juice, and then the gastric pro-tein-B_{12} complex must pass to a specific part of the small intestine (the terminal ileum), where specialized cells permit its absorption into the bloodstream and delivery to the bone marrow.

In PA patients it is the stomach that has been called "the villain of the piece." It is now believed that owing to a chronic inflammation of the stomach lining (gastritis) resulting from an autoimmune reaction—that is, antibodies in the patient attacking his own secretory cells in the stomach—the patient with PA is unable to produce the gastric protein necessary for B_{12} binding and absorption. Inadequate production of red cells or anemia results from this deficiency, and, because parts of the spinal cord also require B_{12} for normal functioning, these patients also develop tingling in the hands and feet, weakness, lack of coordination, and other defects of motor and sensory function that contribute to the incapacitation and ultimate death of the victim.

In the latter part of the nineteenth century and early twentieth century, it was recognized that good nutrition had something to do with blood formation but only in the vaguest way. It was quite natural to include amenia as part of the overall body wasting that was seen in starvation states, for example. The anemias themselves, were specifically classified into two types: primary and secondary. The latter included those that could be directly related to causes such as blood loss or the action of certain toxins on the bone marrow. The primary anemias included all those of unknown or uncertain causes, including PA. In such cases, good diet was ordinarily recommended as part of the treatment, but not as a specific remedy. The term "vitamine" itself was not coined until 1905, and the connection between vitamins and blood formation would have to await the passage of several decades.

Having set the scene for the first breakthroughs in our understanding and treatment of PA, we must introduce three of the major protagonists of this episode which began nearly three quarters of a century after Addison's first description. These were a pathologist working in upstate New York and two Boston internists who had become interested in disorders of the blood.

In 1921, when George Hoyt Whipple, then forty-three, assumed the deanship of the newly formed medical school at the University of Rochester, he had already established himself as a formidable experimental pathologist.[1] A ninth-generation New Englander, the rangy New Hampshireman was the third physician in his family in a direct line from his grandfather. He was also a graduate of the prestigious Johns Hopkins Medical School in Baltimore. At the time of his move to Rochester, he was already involved in the study of blood formation, and had come to this by way of an interest in bile.

Years before, his curiosity had been stimulated by a report that chloroform poisoning in dogs had resulted in liver damage and the appearance of bile pigments in the blood (jaundice). Perhaps the memory of his own bout of jaundice as a fourteen-year-old was a further spur. In any event, he began to study the secretion of bile in dogs surgically manipulated in such a way as to enable him to collect and measure the amounts of bile produced through an abdominal wall fistula (a surgically created channel between the gallbladder and exterior).

While at the University of California in San Francisco, in the post preceding his move to Rochester, Whipple, in 1916, noticed that these surgical procedures often resulted in emaciation of his chronically studied dogs. He found that both their general condition and the production of bile could be improved by the feeding of pig liver. It dawned upon Whipple and his associates that, since bile production was in large part dependent on the result of red cell hemoglobin breakdown, perhaps the liver feeding had somthing to do with the production of hemoglobin, that is, the red blood cells themselves.

It was this consideration that led Whipple to embark on a series of investigations—ultimately, twenty-one in all—in which the effects of feeding various foodstuffs on restoring normal blood hemoglobin and red cell counts would be observed in dogs made chronically anemic through bleeding. By the time he had reached Rochester, Whipple had perfected this model. He and his associates had developed a cross strain of bull terriers and Dalmatian coach hounds suitable in size and disposition for these prolonged experiments. These were all shipped to Rochester when Whipple made his move. After making the dogs anemic through bleeding, Whipple would then feed them a special diet of "salmon bread," a concoction which included flour, bran and tomatoes as well as salmon. With this diet, the time course for the regeneration of the erythrocytes and hemoglobin could be predicted. By adding various other foods to the salmon bread diet, Whipple could determine any additional salutary effect on blood regeneration. Liver seemed to be the most effective substance in correcting the anemia of Whipple's dogs.

News of Whipple's experiments with bleeding-induced anemia and the effects of various dietary elements upon it reached Boston, where Dr. George R. Minot was particularly receptive.[2] Minot's family background was even more impressive medically than Whipple's. His father was a prominent Boston physician; several other relatives, all Harvard trained, had made their marks in Boston medical circles; and his great grandfather had been Dr. James Jackson, a Harvard professor who had helped found both the Massachusetts General Hospital and the *New England Journal of Medicine*.

What especially equipped Minot for the task ahead, however, was his interest in blood disease—he had spent two years at Johns Hopkins studying with the leaders of the fledgling specialty—and his own personal medical history. In 1921, six years after his return to Boston from Baltimore, he had developed diabetes mellitus. In the preinsulin era, it was only the strictest adherence to a most rigid dietary regimen that enabled his survival. When insulin became available in 1923, he was one of the first to take it. But the influence of dietary factors on his psyche had become indelible.

As already stated, there had been some vague thoughts circulating for years about the possible effects of dietary inadequacy in anemia. For pernicious anemia, however, this was only one of several causative possibilities entertained by physicians in the early 1920s, and a minor one at that. Following the great bacteriological discoveries of the preceding Pasteur-Koch-Ehrlich era, there was a great tendency to ascribe an infectious etiology to PA as well as many other diseases that would later be shown to result from other causes. Some thought the anemia was the result of a toxin acting on the bone marrow to prevent the production of red cells. Others thought that excessive destruction of red cells was the cause— a hemolytic anemia. These patients were indeed jaundiced, and it was later shown (1956) that many red cell precursors did die in the bone marrow releasing their pigments into the bloodstream.

Given the lack of any true understanding of the disease, treatments at the time were random and poorly substantiated. Arsenic was a popular "remedy." Removal of the spleen in severe cases was attempted. Finally blood transfusions were administered when they became available.

Minot's gravitation toward the dietary approach was not totally an idiosyncratic one based on his personal experiences. By this time, vitamins were "in the air." Physicians were learning that diseases such as beri-beri, scurvy, and pellagra could be remedied by proper nutritional management. And now there was Whipple and his dogs and their strongly positive response to liver. A visit to Rochester in 1922–23 by Minot to investigate some aspects of insulin research included a discussion of anemia with Whipple. This, no doubt, strengthened his resolve to investigate PA in this way.

To assist him in these clinical studies beginning in 1925, Minot, then forty, selected a man seven years his junior to help him. William Parry Murphy was the antithesis of the patrician Minot.[3] His background and character also belied his name. Far from the popular conception of the natural outgoing Irishman, the mild-mannered self-effacing Murphy was not even Catholic. He was born in Stoughton, Wisconsin and was the son of a Congregational minister. He moved to Oregon with the family as a young man and, after receiving his bachelor's degree from the University of Oregon, taught high school mathematics and physics in Portland in order to finance his first year of medical school at the University of Oregon.

But his heart was set on Harvard. In Portland he continued to receive copies of a newspaper on which he had worked as a boy back in Wisconsin. In one of these he noticed as a filler article an announcement that Dean Briggs from Harvard was about to visit Portland to give the baccalaureate address at Reed College. Murphy worked up his courage and in an uncharacteristically brash move called Briggs upon the latter's arrival to request an interview. They met at the Portland YMCA, where Murphy made known his desire to attend Harvard Medical School—on a full scholarship because he had no money.

"Well, that's interesting," Briggs replied. "I happen to be chairman of the scholarship committee." After a few more words he informed Murphy that he would recommend him for a scholarship for the next term and that "the Committee has never turned down my recommendations."

Murphy, to say the least, was gratified but unaware at the time that only a year before a new fellowship had become available at Harvard following the death of a wealthy Bostonian. The only provision was that it be awarded to one with the same family name as the benefactor, William Stanislaus Murphy.

It was not all the "luck of the Irish," though. Murphy was an excellent student and remembered by his contemporaries as one of the best house officers at the Peter Bent Brigham Hospital in Boston. When he finished his residency, he was invited to join the group practice of several internists including George Minot.

As Minot and Murphy embarked upon their study of liver in PA, they were not the first to use this dietary supplement. A few years before, in 1923, at the University of Iowa some physicians noted moderate improvement following this treatment in PA but considered liver only part of the dietary supportive treatment for the disease. They continued to stress the need for arsenic and iron therapy as well. Even earlier, in 1916, Whipple himself had missed the boat when one of his assistants at the University of California, Charles W. Hooper, hit upon the idea that PA might be due to a specific nutritional deficiency. He tried liver extract with success in six PA patients but never followed up on this with more extensive testing.

Why did Minot and Murphy succeed where the others failed? To begin with, over three quarters of patients with PA were known to have one or more unexplained spontaneous remissions as part of the natural course of the disease. For a time the disease would relent before completing its fatal course. It was often difficult to separate these unpredictable favorable turns of the disease from the truly beneficial effects of any therapy. Furthermore, when liver had been tried in the past, it was often given halfheartedly and with no quantitative emphasis. Ultimately Minot and Murphy were often feeding a half pound of liver or more daily to these patients whose desire for all food was often nil.

Whereas Hooper had not pushed hard enough to follow up on his results in the face of the prevailing skepticism and others, such as those in Iowa, were not quite as perceptive as they might have been, Minot was unrelenting in his determination to see his project followed through in every aspect.

His attention to detail later became legendary. One admirer recalled, "No letter ever went unanswered; a note from him, if not acknowledged in twenty-four hours, was usually followed by another, asking if it had been received. His secretary was once handed a notice to put up on the board. A penciled spot at the top of the paper, surrounded by a circle, was indicated by an arrow from a written directive: 'Put thumbtack here.'" It was this kind of drive that was essential for success.

Murphy, also interested in diseases of the blood, was intelligent, hardworking, and uncomplaining. He was the ideal partner for the enterprise. At the time the work began, Minot was chief of the medical service at Boston's Huntington Memorial Hospital, dedicated to the care of cancer patients. Murphy, in private practice, was an attending physician at the Peter Bent Brigham Hospital next door. It was he who provided the access to the PA patients, supervised their diets, and oversaw the blood work that was essential to evaluate the effects of the treatment.

One final factor made their work easier: the use of the reticulocyte count. Reticulocytes, so named because of the filamentous network that appears within them on proper staining, are young red cells. Their percentage among the total number of erythrocytes increases relatively early after successful therapy, long before the total number of red cells or the hemoglobin content of the blood show any improvement. Years before, Minot and others had detected the usefulness of this phenomenon as an early sign of increased bone marrow activity with the successful treatment of various anemias. Although the hallmark of PA is the megaloblast, a large juvenile red cell in arrested development, it was through counting the reticulocytes that an early effect could be demonstrated. This was critical in light of the widespread reluctance of hospital authorities to deviate from the more conventional treatments in PA, especially blood transfusions in the more seriously ill.

Minot's and Murphy's enthusiasm was certainly not shared by their superiors or others on the scene. Dr. Henry Christian, the chief of medicine at the Brigham, agreed to let them do the work as long as the patients were in no danger of dying. The medical house officers (interns and residents) wanted to gain experience in administering blood transfusions, the best palliative treatment at the time, and they eagerly awaited this opportunity with the PA patients.

Murphy's first patient was admitted to the hospital and the forced feeding with liver begun. By midnight of the fourth day, Murphy found that the reticulocyte count, often hovering at about 1 percent in PA patients, had risen to 4 percent in his patient. Believing this a sign of response, he refused to transfuse the patient. Murphy slept poorly that night. He knew the medical residents ate breakfast at seven and would soon thereafter be making their ward rounds. He rose early and rushed to the hospital to head them off, although "the thought crossed my mind that I might find him dead." As Murphy reached the bedside, the patient sat up and querulously inquired, "Aren't we going to have any breakfast?" Murphy then felt assured that they were on the right track.

In the August 14, 1926, issue of the *Journal of the American Medical Association*, Minot and Murphy published the results of their special diet in forty-five PA patients treated for up to six months.[4] This landmark of research clearly demonstrated the efficacy of liver. Throughout the world physicians and patients marveled at the life-saving miracle, and numerous honors were bestowed upon the two Boston physicians.

Ironically, a key element of ignorance was essential to their success. The cause of the anemia in Whipple's dogs was, at the time, understood neither by Whipple nor by Minot and Murphy. It would not be until 1936 that Whipple would determine that the anemia secondary to chronic blood loss was due to depletion of the body's iron stores and treatable by iron supplements. Since iron therapy had already been tried in PA without effect before the time of Minot and Murphy's studies, Whipple's success with liver in his dogs might have been disregarded by the Boston pair had they known this. It turns out that liver contains large amounts of *both* iron and vitamin B_{12}, so much of the latter that, despite the loss of the binding protein in the stomachs of the PA patients, the mass effect of the B_{12} given was enough to ensure sufficient absorption and clinical response. It was the iron in the liver, of course, that was the effective agent in Whipple's dogs.

As the world celebrated the results of the liver treatment in PA, a better understanding of the cause of the disease awaited the posing of a critical question. This was supplied approximately two years after Minot and Murphy's report by one of Minot's own assistants, a tall gangling twenty-nine-year-old research associate at the Thorndike Memorial Laboratory of Boston City Hospital, where Minot had succeeded Francis W. Peabody, its first director.

William B. Castle had begun his interest in PA many years earlier as a sophomore medical student at Harvard. He had failed a course in hematology and in the makeup examination had been questioned about anemias by the head of the Thorndike, Dr. Peabody.

The success of Minot and Murphy rekindled Castle's interest in PA. The question that intrigued him was: Why don't normal persons need a half pound of liver daily in order to prevent the development of pernicious anemia? The clue seemed to lie in the stomach, which for many years had been recognized as being atrophic in patients with the disease. Was there something in PA sufferers that was missing that was present in the stomachs of normal individuals?

Castle later described the simple but definitive approach he

applied to answering this question. "The experimental procedure consisted of two consecutive periods of ten days or
more during which daily reticulocyte counts were made. During the first period of ten days the patient received 200
g(rams) of rare hamburg steak [lean beef muscle] daily as the
only source of animal protein. There was no increase in the
number of reticulocytes."

It was the second part of the protocol that was so critical
and startling even in recollection today. Castle himself would
then eat a portion of hamburger steak and one hour later pass
a tube through his nose and into the stomach to collect the
partially digested contents and gastric juice. These he would
allow to incubate several hours until liquefaction of the meat
had occurred before delivering the contents to a PA patient
through another nasogastric tube.*

The PA patients thus treated showed a response: their reticulocyte count began to climb, and their anemia was corrected as treatment continued.[5]

As the experiments progressed, in subsequent years the
source of normal gastric juice became a series of medical students Castle dubbed "gastric juicers," who were paid for their
services.

Castle found that only a combination of the normal gastric
juice and the "hamburg" steak was effective. Either given
alone was useless in eliciting the desired response. One might
wonder, in retrospect, why he used Hamburger steak rather
than liver, as was done by Minot and Murphy. He has written
that at the time meat and liver "naively" struck him as similar.
Of course there is also B_{12} in hamburger steak, although not
so plentiful as in liver.

Thus two factors were distinguished by Castle. One, contained in the proper diet, he called the "extrinsic factor," and
one, found in normal gastric contents, he called the "intrinsic

*In the current era of informed consent and hospitals' human medical re-
search committees, one might well speculate about the chances he might
have in getting such a program under way today.

factor." These would later be identified as B_{12} and the gastric binding protein.

A number of subsequent investigators, most of them biochemists or other laboratory "bench workers," added the final touches to the picture with the isolation and identification of B_{12}, or cyanocobalamin (it contains cobalt). The gastric protein was described and its interaction with B_{12} clarified. Tests were devised to diagnose PA more accurately and to differentiate it from its impersonators. The autoimmune nature of the disorder was determined. An injectable form of B_{12} requiring only monthly administration made management over the long term considerably easier for these patients and was only partly vitiated by the fact that many unscrupulous or ignorant practitioners gave many of their patients routine B_{12} "shots" when they were totally unnecessary.

None of these later developments, however, had the profound effects on medical science as did the initial work of Whipple, Minot, Murphy, and Castle. Hematology was transformed almost overnight from the passive pathological study of blood slides to a dynamic physiological evaluation of the body's blood-forming system. The stranglehold of bacteriological thinking on medical researchers seeking the causes of disease was broken. Clinical research in the United States received a major stimulus, and developing specialists in other medical fields attempted to achieve results at the bedside in ways similar to those of these pioneer investigators.

It was not surprising that in 1934 the Nobel Committee chose to honor Whipple, Minot, and Murphy for their work on the dietary treatment of anemia, although many have felt that Castle was equally deserving of this honor. The biochemists and other laboratory workers who also contributed importantly to our knowledge and treatment of PA have been even more neglected by the public, and remain nameless and faceless to the vast majority of us.

More important than the distribution of accolades, however, have been the effects of these discoveries on ourselves. At the Nobel ceremony in 1934, the presentor estimated that since the time of Minot and Murphy's discovery, between fifteen and twenty thousand lives had been saved in the United States alone. Think of the countless thousands more worldwide between then and now.

The potential victims of PA and their families owe an incalculable debt to the perception and persistence of Minot and Murphy and those who followed them. To this day, their accomplishment continues to permeate our routine daily existence. After all, who among us has not heard a concerned mother at one time or another admonish her children, "Eat your liver. It's good for you!"

From Trench Warfare to War on Cancer

The Development of Chemotherapy for Malignant Disease

"As we looked to our left, we saw a thick, yellowish-green cloud veiling the sky like a cloud of vapor. We were already affected by asphyxiating fumes. I had the impression that I was looking through green glasses. At the same time, I felt the action of the gas upon my respiratory system; it burned my throat, caused pains in my chest, and made breathing all but impossible. I spat blood and suffered from dizziness. We all thought we were lost."[1]

This was how a French army doctor recalled the second battle of Ypres when, on April 22, 1915, the German army introduced gas warfare to the Western Front. The chlorine gas was driven by the winds close to the ground over the Allied lines as a five-foot high, four-mile-long cloud. There were more than five thousand casualties from the first attack alone.

Soon the Allies afforded their soldiers protection with gas masks, which were protective not only against chlorine but against its successor, phosgene, another lung irritant. This led to the introduction of a new type of poison gas in 1917, the most efficient of all the noxious vapors that the wartime chemists seemed capable of devising. This was a vesicant (blister-forming) gas, and Ypres again was the testing ground when it made its deadly debut against the Allied troops.

An official name for the new agent was "Yperite," commemorating the place where it was introduced. Many soldiers called it "hot stuff," which it certainly was. But the most common name that has come down to us derived from its smell, which resembled garlic or, more often, a common table condiment. Hence the name "mustard gas." Not only did the new gas irritate the linings of the lungs, causing pneumonia and bronchitis; it was equally active against the membranes of the eyes and nose. The oily substance was also rapidly absorbed by the skin. There, after a short interval, it would result in blisters which would grow in size for days and heal only slowly. Particularly insidious among its properties was the ability of mustard gas to inflict similar injuries on those who did not come in direct contact with it, but had only touched garments or equipment on which it had come to rest days before.

Mustard gas became the most successful of all these noxious agents. The memory of its debilitating triumphs on the battlefield more than seventy years ago survived even to the extent of recommending it more recently to the Iraqis in their frustrating stalemate with the Iranians along their borders. By the end of World War I, mustard gas and its cousins in the chemical armamentarium of the combatants had accounted for at least 1.3 million casualties on both sides of the conflict. About ninety-one thousand had died acutely; many thousands more lingered on as respiratory cripples for the decades between the two great wars.

Yet from all this misery and destruction, great good was to come. The first evidence we have of mustard gas's potential use as a chemotherapeutic agent came from a study performed in 1919 by the Krumbhaars, a pair of investigators at the University of Pennsylvania.[2] During the First World War, it had been found that in about a quarter of the soldiers exposed to mustard gas, following an initial rise in the white blood cell count, there was often a precipitous fall. When the counts were significantly depressed below normal, the prognosis for the patient worsened considerably, apparently owing to a lack of resistance to infection in the absence of sufficient numbers of these protective cells. Since these findings were not uniformly present in surviving military men who were often in various stages of recovery, the Krumbhaars examined the bone marrows of those who had died and demonstrated that there was truly a depression of blood cell formation in such cases.

In the decades that followed, there was little research activity to follow up on this seminal study. There seemed little need to investigate the effect of poison gas after "the war to end all wars." However, by the late 1930s, the Japanese had overrun Manchuria, the Nazis had taken over Germany, and fascism was firmly ensconced in Italy and Spain as well. The maintenance of peaceful international relations once again became seriously in doubt. With the possibility of armed conflict once again a concern in Washington, D.C., memories of the devastating effects of gas warfare were revived. Although the Geneva Protocol on Gas Warfare had outlawed this in 1925, no one was betting that the ban would prevent a reintroduction of poison gas during any future hostilities, and stockpiling of the deadly materials began in secret.

In 1942, a contract was signed between Yale University and the Office of Scientific Research and Development of the United States government to investigate chemical warfare agents. The study of mustard gas was assigned to Drs. Louis S. Goodman and Alfred Gilman, pharmacologists, who, with their associates, began to study its effects in animals in order to develop a suitable antidote.[3] Early on, it was found that mustard gas itself was a difficult agent to use in such work because of its extreme reactivity and the inability to dissolve it in fluids for intravenous administration. By substituting a nitrogen molecule for sulfur in the structure, however, the researchers were able to proceed with their animal experimentation more easily.

It soon became apparent that those tissues with the most proliferative activity under normal conditions were precisely those that were most affected by the poison. This included the skin, the linings of the gastrointestinal tract, and especially the bone marrow and lymphoid tissues where blood cells were formed.

At about this time, Dr. Thomas Dougherty was working in the Department of Anatomy at Yale, studying the effects of estrogens on mouse leukemias. He learned from Goodman and Gilman about the experiments they were conducting on the effects of nitrogen mustard on the lymphoid tissue of rabbits. Dougherty had one mouse in which an experimental lymphoma (tumor of lymphoid tissue) had been transplanted and which had grown to such an enormous size that it had dwarfed the rest of the animal. Such tumors often did this, leading to the death of the recipient within a period of about three weeks following implantation.

Dougherty and his colleagues decided to give some nitrogen mustard to their laboratory mouse, and after two doses the tumor began to soften and decrease in size. Eventually it could no longer even be palpated. Treatment was stopped, and after about a month the tumor began to reappear. Subsequent treatments had diminishing effectiveness, but there was no doubt about the results of the treatment: the mouse had survived for a remarkable eighty-four days postimplantation because of the nitrogen mustard therapy. This particular type of experimental lymphoma—C3HEDT or the Gardner tumor, after Dougherty's colleague who had developed it— became a standard testing tumor for anticancer drugs in many laboratories in the years that followed.

As Dougherty recalled years later, the choice of the C3HEDT lymphoma was very fortuitous. In many other mouse lymphomas later tried, the effect of nitrogen mustard was much less marked, and in most mouse leukemias no effect at all was seen with nitrogen mustard. He wrote to Gilman, "I have often thought that if we had by accident chosen one of these leukemias in which there was absolutely no therapeutic effect, we might possibly have dropped the whole project."[4]

The unpredictability of response to nitrogen mustard by various tumors was an early lesson learned by these investigators and would apply to other agents that would later be developed. They also soon learned that while they tried to eradicate cancerous tissue within the host, the normal bone marrow might also be dangerously suppressed, just as it was in those World War I fatalities from gassing. Both aspects of chemotherapy for cancer continue to plague those involved in the development of new agents.

The success of further mouse experiments encouraged the Yale group to attempt the treatment of human cancer with nitrogen mustard. Their first subject was a forty-eight-year-old man in the terminal stages of lymphosarcoma, which was no longer responsive to X-ray therapy. The enlarging tumor masses involved the chest, armpits, face, neck, and chin. Venous drainage from the head and neck was impeded, and the face and upper chest were swollen and blue. The patient could hardly chew or swallow, and breathing itself was threatened as the tumor masses engulfed his airways. A tracheostomy set was kept in readiness at the bedside for emergency use should the windpipe be cut off completely.

As with that first mouse, following the nitrogen mustard, the patient showed a remarkable response with the tumor masses melting away to the extent that, within two weeks, they were no longer palpable. With no previous experience with dosage requirements that would cause tumor regression without suppressing normal blood cell production, the doctors at Yale, as elsewhere in these initial therapeutic trials, had to feel their way. This first patient suffered a severe reduction of all his blood elements following his treatment with nitrogen mustard. When he died three months after the start of therapy, it was believed that it was this serious side effect of the drug that had led to his demise rather than the original tumor which had remained greatly reduced in size.

In May 1946, the results of the initial trials in sixty-seven patients at New Haven and cooperating units in Salt Lake City, Boston, and Portland, Oregon, were reported in the *Journal of the American Medical Association*.[5] This multicenter trial set the pattern for future research of this kind in attempts to accumulate sufficient numbers of appropriate patients to determine the effectiveness of different therapeutic protocols. Among this group were not only patients with lymphosarcoma, but those with Hodgkin's disease and various leukemias. Despite the problems already mentioned, it was clear that a new era in the treatment of cancer had arrived.

Prior to the introduction of chemotherapy, treatment of

cancer was limited to surgery and radiation treatment (X rays or radium). When localized and reasonably small, some cancers could be completely removed by surgical means. Unfortunately, many cancers spread beyond the bounds of curable extirpation by the time they are discovered and brought to the surgeon's attention. Soon after their discovery by Roentgen in 1895, X rays were found useful in the treatment of skin cancers but later abandoned because of problems with skin burns and proper dose determination. By 1922, however, at the International Congress of Otology in Paris, six cases of advanced laryngeal cancer successfully treated with X rays were presented. Radium, another source of radiation, was used in needle implants only a few years after its discovery by the Curies in 1898. Other radioactive substances discovered since then have also been useful in the treatment of cancer but, like X ray therapy, limited by the intolerance of the normal cells in the body to excessive radiation.

The availability of nitrogen mustard enabled physicians to treat certain neoplasms that were beyond the help of surgery or no longer amenable to radiation therapy.

Nitrogen mustard was not the first drug ever used in the treatment of cancer. In preceding decades certain drugs such as colchicine, arsenic, and urethane were observed to have some mild antitumor activity and were so employed. Other new approaches to cancer therapy—hormones and more recently, experimental immunological techniques with monoclonal antibodies—have been added to the potential treatment of this dreaded group of diseases that we call cancer. The striking success of nitrogen mustard, however, opened the door to a therapeutic approach with agents that seemed specifically designed for this purpose and no others in clinical medicine.

How do they work? In various ways, apparently. Originally it was thought the effects, therapeutic and toxic, of nitrogen mustard were related to the fact that, following contact with body surfaces, mustard gas forms hydrochloric acid. Later, more sophisticated research showed that nitrogen mustard acts on cancer cells by alkylation—they bind chemically with the DNA within the rapidly proliferating cancer cells and thereby prevent their continued replication. Other alkylating agents with similar actions to nitrogen mustard were to emerge from the laboratory and prove, in many instances, superior to it. Other chemotherapeutic agents now in common use work quite differently and often have emerged under circumstances no less unique than those leading to the discovery of their forerunner.

Nutritional research led to the development of a new class of such drugs. As far back as 1944 investigators at Mt. Sinai Hospital in New York had reported that folic acid, a dietary constituent necessary for the normal formation of red blood cells, inhibited tumor growths (experimental sarcomas) in mice. However, when a pioneer in cancer research, Dr. Sidney Farber, and his colleagues in Boston attempted to use such knowledge in the treatment of childhood leukemia, they found that the condition of the patients actually *worsened* with the administration of folic acid. This led to their using antifolates with beneficial effect.[6] Such antimetabolites are still useful in the management of certain malignancies.

Oncologists have also benefited from attempts to find new antibiotics. Actinomycin, developed as an antituberculosis drug, has proved much more effective in a number of neoplastic diseases. Daunorubicin, a potent antileukemic agent, had similar origins.

Folk medicine provided a derivative of the common periwinkle plant. Extracts of periwinkle had been used for more than a century for treating diabetes in places such as the Philippines, South Africa, and India. A Canadian endocrinologist was stimulated by such knowledge to administer extracts to rabbits to verify this. The blood sugar in these animals did not fall, and the rabbits all died from overwhelming infection. The cause of this problem was found to be a drop in the white cell count owing to bone morrow suppression. Vinblastine, a new anticancer agent, was the final result.

Immunology research, in a somewhat indirect way, made an important contribution early on. In 1953, it was shown that guinea pig serum caused regression of tumors in mice and rats. The factor isolated that was responsible for this effect was an enzyme, l-asparaginase, which became an important part of the therapeutic regimen in the treatment of acute lymphocytic leukemia in children. More recently, the potential of monoclonal antibodies has been recognized as a new immunological approach for the early detection and treatment of cancer and is under active investigation at a number of centers throughout the country.

One of the most recent additions to the list of useful drugs has a history of chance discovery rivaling in serendipity all the many others discovered this way in the past. Dr. Barnet Rosenberg and his associates in the Biophysics Department at Michigan State University were trying to determine the effects of electrical fields on the growth of bacteria. They reported an unexpected result of their experiments in *Nature* in 1965.[7] They had found that after creating an electrical field within a chamber containing *E. coli,* they had caused a clearing in the appearance of the solution; that is, decrease in the turbidity (a reflection of bacterial population density.) The turbidity was restored upon elimination of the electrical field. This effect could be repeatedly reproduced by the application of voltages across the culture chamber. During the periods of clearing, they noticed under the microscope that the *E. coli* were elongated and in an arrested stage of growth. Normal cell division resumed once the current was turned off.

In the original design of the experiment, Rosenberg had elected to use platinum for the electrodes because of its presumed chemical inertness. But it was hardly inert as far as the bacteria were concerned because the platinum entering the solution was inhibiting their reproduction. Cisplatin, especially useful in testicular and ovarian carcinomas, has resulted from this chance observation.

The application of these very diversified drugs, collectively called chemotherapeutic agents, especially when combined with surgery, radiation, and occasionally hormonal therapy, has revolutionized the approach to cancer treatment. It has relieved the unrelenting picture of gloom and death that was the lot of almost all cancer victims as recently as the 1960s.

Nitrogen mustard rarely effected cures, and frequently the currently used agents only ameliorate rather than eliminate the diseases for which they are prescribed. Yet the earlier tentative reports of two-year survivals, then five-year survivals, then ten-year survivals have finally blossomed into declarations of complete remissions—cures—from the physicians and surgeons who have devoted their careers to this aspect of medicine.

I vividly recall a time in the early 1960s when my colleagues and I lined up to donate blood in the hopeless cause of prolonging the life of a friend's severely anemic eighteen-month-old boy who was dying of acute leukemia. Yet today it is the childhood leukemias and others of the most agressive cancers, those often affecting children or young adults, that are the most amenable to cure. Over the last twenty years about a dozen tumors that were once uniformly fatal are now curable in most patients: uterine choriocarcinoma, acute lymphocytic leukemia and sarcomas in children, Hodgkin's disease, other lymphomas, testicular cancer in young men. Ovarian cancer can be helped significantly in a number of cases.

Combinations of surgery and radiation with chemotherapy, as noted above, have been recognized as an important element of success along with recognition of the roles of environmental factors and personal behavior such as cigarette smoking. Such satisfactions, however, are tempered by the realization that cancer still remains the second leading cause of death in the United States—ranking behind cardiovascular disease—and that this rank is related mainly to the fact that the most common cancers (lung, breast, and colon) are often the least responsive to chemotherapy and often beyond the ability of all types of therapy to obtain cures by the time the malignancy is discovered. Oftentimes, an effective cancer drug is also the cause of severe toxic side effects. Thus the constant search for new more effective and safer drugs along with innovative other approaches to prevent or cure these diseases.

While failure often seems to be the handmaiden to success in such endeavors, those who have been intimately involved in the progress that has been made cannot help but be poignantly reminded of what the beginnings of cancer chemotherapy has meant to them. This was conveyed in part of a letter one of these investigators, Thomas Dougherty of Yale, wrote to Alfred Gilman almost twenty years after their original experience with nitrogen mustard in New Haven.

"You might be interested to know that I still have practically all the blood films, bone marrows and the sections of the organs, etc. of both mice and men treated at that time. I have thrown out a few blood films, but could not bring myself to throw this part of my life completely in the ash can."[8]

Sparks

Life-Giving Electricity

It was San Francisco in the summer of 1958. Mr. Valerian, as
we shall call him, had entered Mount Zion Hospital for what
he realized might be the last time. For the major portion of his
life, he had indeed been fortunate. He had arrived in the
United States many years before, a penniless Hungarian immigrant, but had managed to achieve the American dream.
He had prospered in business; he had married the woman of
his choice and raised a family that adored him; and, at seventy
years of age, he had looked forward to spending his remaining days in comfortable retirement, doting upon his numerous
grandchildren.

Several months before this hospital admission, however, his
existence had been blighted by the onset of ill health. One
day, while visiting a friend in the hospital, he suddenly lost
consciousness and fell to the floor. A house doctor rushed to
his side and found that his pulse was only twenty beats per
minute. What went wrong?

In Mr Valerian's case, the "wiring" between the upper and
lower chambers of the heart had been disrupted, and the ventricles, lacking reception of impulses from above, were beating
at their own intrinsically slow rate.* In the presence of this

---

*Each part of the heart has its own intrinsic or characteristic rate at which it
will beat if not stimulated from some other part of the heart with a more

heart block, whenever these rates happened to fall to excessively low levels, the attacks would recur. Within a few months'
time, the episodes of unconsciousness with seizures had become frighteningly common. Yet, despite the severity and frequency of these spells, Mr. Valerian managed somehow to
maintain the lively wit, charm, and equanimity that seemed to
defy the hopelessness of his condition.

At the time of his admission to the hospital, Mr. Valerian's
heart muscle had become increasingly resistant to the acceler-
ating effects of the medications that had been administered to
him, first by mouth and later intravenously, in hopes of maintaining heart rates high enough to maintain adequate perfusion of his brain. While he rested in bed, for the most part his
heart rate was slow but acceptable. Then, several times a day
the rate would relentlessly decrease until it was insufficient to
maintain consciousness and another attack would occur. Imminent death was the result in most patients reaching this
stage of their illness. The heart would often go into complete
arrest, and no restoration of function would be obtained even
with the most heroic of emergency measures, including the
direct intracardiac administration of potent medications by insertion of a needle through the chest wall. But in Mr. Valerian's case, the clinical course was quite unusual and, in a

---

rapid intrinsic rate. The ventricles, the muscular lower chambers of the
heart that propel blood either to the lungs (right ventricle) or to the rest of
the body (left ventricle) have a basic rate of only thirty to fifty beats per
minute, at times less. In most people, such rates are too slow to maintain
normal activity. When the rate begins to fall below forty, insufficient blood
supplied to the brain may result in loss of consciousness, often with attendant seizures. Fortunately, in one of the upper chambers of the heart, the
right atrium, a nubbin of excitable conduction tissue called the sinus node is
present to drive, through its branching, the rest of the heart at rates we
recognize as normal (seventy to one hundred beats per minute). The impulses spread through the right and left atria, converge on another node
(the atrioventricular), which then, in continuation of the electrical pathway,
activates the right and left ventricles through their respective [bundle]
branches of conduction fibers.

way, singularly perverse. His heart refused to respond to the chronic administration of medications, but, somehow, he had survived dozens of fainting attacks over the course of several weeks. He lived in limbo, in a sort of medical purgatory in which his condition would neither improve nor terminate once and for all.

At the time of his hospital admission, the plan was to withdraw the routine oral administration of all medications which had previously been given every three or four hours in hopes of forestalling attacks. Treatment would now be given only for the attacks as they occurred. In this manner, without the constant exposure to the presence of drugs in the blood, his heart muscle might gradually regain responsiveness to their effects for future management. The risk of doing this was not considered excessive. Although he had already developed poor responsiveness to the drugs, he had also demonstrated a remarkable capacity to recover from the attacks and besides, what else was there to do?

He was placed in a centrally located room in order to be as accessible as possible to all staff on call.* He was to remain in bed with a family member or nursing assistant in constant attendance. An intravenous line was in place to permit rapid administration of medications as necessary. With the onset of an attack, the telephone operator would be notified immediately and announce a prearranged code message over the loudspeaker system. The first physician to reach Mr. Valerian would be responsible for intravenous infusion of the medication necessary for termination of the attack.

The plan as outlined proceeded for two weeks. The house staff responded, the attacks were terminated but did not decrease in number or severity. Each time, as the convulsions ceased and consciousness returned, Mr. Valerian would look up and smile wanly. "Well what do you know, doc? I made it again."

---

*At this time the installation of coronary units or critical care units in hospitals had not yet become routine.

Neither the patient nor his physicians believed it could go on much longer. After three weeks without improvement, the routine oral medications were resumed with no resultant change in the frequency or severity of the attacks. The trial had failed; his heart was just as unresponsive as ever. With no improvement, it was impossible to discharge him from the hospital, and the emergency calls continued unabated. As the sense of frustration increased, another plan of action was developed. By this time, I had been assigned to the case—in my capacity as an intern—to assist the attending physician, Dr. John J. Sampson, and one of the junior cardiologists on staff who had become increasingly involved, Dr. Herman Uhley.[1]

Uhley had already been recognized as something of a "whiz kid." An ingenious tinkerer in electronics, the frail-looking "four-eyed" scholar, always with an incipient self-effacing smile, could easily then—and even now— conjure up the impression of a local high school's senior-class "brain." He was probably one of the first civilians to own a walkie-talkie, at least in San Francisco, and during the course of the day he delighted in communicating with another lark-loving staffman of similar bent without the benefit of telephone lines.

My own awakening interest in cardiology had been noticed by Uhley. One of my earliest recollections of him is his emergence from the morgue one day as I just happened to pass by. "Hey, Al. Come over here, I want to show you something." And like a conspiratorial adolescent, he revealed his treasure to me.

Uhley had learned that conduction tissue would dramatically stain with a common iodine-containing liquid (Lugol's solution), whereas the ordinary heart muscle surrounding it would not. He opened the heart whose interior he had swabbed with Lugol's, and there it was: a golden-brown thread running through the cavity of the left ventricle and clearly standing out from the remaining heart and fibrous tissue—the left bundle branch. I had read a bit about this major activating switch of the heart's electrical circuit and even seen it diagrammed in many texts and on the blackboard. I had often diagnosed "left bundle branch block" on electrocardiograms.

And here it was, visible to the naked eye, touchable! It actually "existed!" If anyone at Mother Zion could help poor Mr. Valerian, I thought, it would have to be Herman Uhley.

Cardiac pacing was in its infancy at the time, and no standard equipment or procedures were in effect. In Boston, electrical impulses had been applied externally to the chest wall by Dr. Paul Zoll to shock extra beats into the excessively slow-beating heart. Uhley's idea was to rig up a device for stimulating the heart from *within*. Using the remains of a friend's old television set, he had constructed an apparatus that developed a small repetitive voltage that could be delivered into the patient's heart. A wire from this would be threaded through a standard cardiac catheter, the bare tip protruding through the end. Dr. Elliot Rapaport, then head of the heart catheterization laboratory at Mount Zion, would introduce the catheter into an arm vein and advance it into the heart, permitting electrical stimulation of the organ internally.

Desperate for any possible successful resolution to the problem, Mr. Valerian and his family agreed to the plan. In the catheterization room, under fluoroscopy, the catheter with its wire was inserted and advanced centrally into the chest and finally into the right ventricle of the heart. The pacemaking apparatus was activated, and for the first time since the onset of his illness Mr. Valerian had a normal heart rate without any recourse to stimulatory cardiac drugs.

He was returned to his room, and all of us were in a state of tentative elation. Would it continue to work? Would the attacks cease completely? What would be the complications? Could we possibly electrocute him?

The patient was "plugged" into the wall outlet next to his bed to receive house current needed for operation of the pacemaker, and we awaited the results. One day, two days, three days passed without a single attack. The private nurses were discharged from the case. No longer were family and friends required to maintain a constant vigil. No code-calls requiring immediate response were breathlessly announced over the loudspeaker system. Now long-term plans were called for in order to ensure proper maintenance of the system. How long could it be kept in place without the risk of infection being introduced through the exposed arm vein? How long would it take for the heart muscle to become responsive once again to the medications one might wish to resume prescribing?

Shortly thereafter, a battery-powered portable external pacemaker, recently developed by Dr. Paul Zoll (see discussion later in this chapter) was shipped from Boston to enable the patient to move about his room freely from time to time. But about a week later, Mr. Valerian obviated the need for any further planning on his behalf. Apparently, awakening in a somewhat confused state that morning, he inadvertently unplugged the cable from the pacemaker as he crossed the room. Losing consciousness, he fell to the floor, striking his head severely. He was discovered by the orderly who was making his routine morning rounds. The cause of death was a massive brain hemorrhage.

Despite the sad ending of this episode, of one thing we could be certain: a promising new treatment for complete heart block had been demonstrated, and the rest of the medical world should be made aware of it. It was at this point that a report was received from the East Coast. Drs. Seymour Furman and John B. Schwedel at Montefiore Hospital in the Bronx had already announced their own success in two patients with an almost identical setup and were about to publish their results in the *New England Journal of Medicine*. They had "beaten us to the punch."[2]

To the nonscientist, at first blush it must seem almost incomprehensible that living beings could have any biological connection with electricity as we ordinarily think about it: light bulbs, toasters, radios, television, and the like. Yet the ancients were well aware of the phenomenon we call electricity as manifested by the charges emitted from torpedo fish (electric rays) and electric catfish. The early Greeks even believed the sting of such fish to be helpful in the treatment of headaches, epilepsy, and other maladies.[3]

The relationship between magnetism and electricity was also recognized at an early date. When fossilized resins such as amber were rubbed, they could attract light objects such as feathers; the Greek word for amber, *electron,* has been retained in its various forms down through the centuries to describe this branch of science. In the latter half of the eighteenth century, especially, interest in the experimentation with electrical phenomena accelerated. Every American schoolchild is taught about Benjamin Franklin's fascination with lightning and electricity and his forays into the atmosphere with his kites to probe such mysteries. A number of other brilliant minds have focused more specifically on bioelectrical phenomena, and many are recalled in the terminology that has developed in relation to them. Volt, ampere, joule, ohm, coulomb, galvanometer, and farad, for example, can be traced back to the likes of Alessandro Volta, André-Marie Ampère, James Prescott Joule, Georg Ohm, Charles Augustin de Coulomb, Luigi Galvani, and Michael Faraday.

Much of the early work along these lines involved the demonstration of electrical excitability of various animal structures. A case in point was an early experiment of Galvani in the eighteenth century in which he demonstrated the contractions of frog leg muscles when stimulated through their nerve supply by electrical current. Recognition of inherent electrical activity within many living tissues—other than such bizarre specimens as the electric eel—came later, mainly because of the minute amounts of electricity generated and the inability of the available instrumentation of the times to detect it. The heart of a mammal, for example, rarely generates electrical impulses in excess of 3/1000 volt, an amount undetectable in the laboratory until relatively recently.

But, in truth, we are all walking conglomerates of thousands of tiny dynamos. There is not the flutter of an eyelid, the rumbling of a gut, the jerk of a knee, the formation of a smile, or, for that matter, an opinion that takes place without the exchange of some charged particles signaling an electrical event within us.

Of all the body's organs, perhaps none has been so dramatically demonstrated to be dependent on its electrical activity as the heart, at least as manifested in clinical medicine. An electrocardiogram is an almost routine test performed on most hospital or office patients, especially those over forty, regardless of the character of the primary complaint. Yet it was not until the end of the nineteenth century that this minute electrical activity could be demonstrated and well into the twentieth century before such measurements could be made routine.

By the end of the nineteenth century, electrical activity in animal hearts, exposed by thoracotomy, had been demonstrated in physiology laboratories. Credit for recording the first cardiac electrical potentials in the intact human being goes to Augustus Désiré Waller (1856–1922), a bumptious brilliant physiologist who was born and received his early education on the Continent but who emigrated in his youth to Great Britain, where he performed a major portion of his work at the University of London and St. Mary's Hospital. It was at the latter institution in 1887 that "I dipped my right hand and left foot into a couple of basins of salt solution which were connected with the two poles of the electrometer and at once had the pleasure of seeing the mercury column pulsate with the pulsation of the heart."[4]

The Lippman electrometer he used consisted of a column of mercury within a glass tube immersed in a solution of dilute sulfuric acid. The electrical discharges from the heart caused a fluctuation of the mercury within the tube and a magnified image of the moving mercury column could be recorded on sensitized recording paper. Although it is hard to comprehend in the light of present knowledge, Waller never recognized the enormous potential of his discovery and expressed doubts as to electrocardiograms—as he dubbed them—ever being useful in clinical investigation, no less routine patient care.

Present at that portentous St. Mary's demonstration of 1887 was a friend of Waller's, the Dutch physician and physiologist Willem Einthoven (1860–1927), who immediately recognized the tremendous possibilities of Waller's discovery. The torch in electrocardiography passed from the flamboyant Waller to the staid Einthoven, who returned to the University of Leyden to grapple with the problem and the possibilities of this new research tool.[5]

At first, he tried continuing work with the capillary electrometer of Lippman, which, although promising at first, soon revealed many deficiencies. It was not sensitive enough; it exhibited too much inertia; it was prey to increased friction from dust particles that inevitably worked their way into the apparatus. A breakthrough in his research then came from a field totally removed from animal or human biology. With the laying of submerged marine telegraph cables in the midnineteenth century, the need for improved instrumentation to receive dispatches became acute. However, the industrial galvanometers available at the time of Einthoven's entrance into the field were too crude and insensitive for the purpose of recording cardiac electrical activity. Efforts had begun by some investigators to improve upon this by developing more sensitive instruments. Einthoven continued this work.

As much a physicist as a physician or physiologist, he adopted and improved the string galvanometer for use in human electrocardiography. Although his prototype machine that housed all the elements of the system was as big as a small Volkswagen, it was extremely accurate and enabled him to lay the groundwork for all future discoveries in the field of electrocardiography. Soon all sorts of cardiac abnormalities—chamber enlargement, insufficiency of coronary blood flow, irregularities of the heartbeat, and, of course, heart block—could be diagnosed with accuracy.

Although his name is known to every physician who ever studied electrocardiography, Einthoven remains, for the most part, a shadowy figure in contemporary minds. In a photograph occasionally reproduced in histories of medicine, he appears in his laboratory, a bald, bearded figure in black, flanked by several assistants, all of them nearly displaced by the enormous bulk of this early instrument of his devising. As indicated above, a major problem confronting Einthoven was to construct a filament fine enough to reflect the tiny electrical currents generated by the heart.

His Rube Goldberg approach to the solution seems totally out of character for a "respectable" scientist. To obtain a fine quartz string, "The tail end of an arrow was attached by an element of quartz to the string of a tightly drawn bow. The quartz was heated and, as it melted, the arrow was released and shot across the room, drawing the quartz into a fine string. At times, the string was picked out of the air when it was held up by currents in the room."[6]

No less notable than his ingenuity and resourcefulness was Einthoven's generosity. Never too good with his hands, he relied greatly on the dexterity and other skills of his laboratory assistant van de Woerd. When Einthoven received a Nobel prize in 1924 for his contributions to electrocardiography, the sum involved was the equivalent of $40,000. Einthoven then began a search for van de Woerd, who had long since retired. When he discovered that his former assistant had died, Einthoven gave half the prize money to two surviving sisters of van de Woerd who had been living in genteel poverty.

A year before, Canadian surgeon Frederick Banting had received a Nobel for the discovery of insulin. Although the committee had included as a corecipient of this honor Banting's superior, John R. McLeod, professor of physiology at the University of Toronto, they had ignored the medical student who had worked so closely with Banting on the project, Charles H. Best. Banting made a point of his disapproval by sharing his half of the award with Best. Although Banting's act of honor and largesse is well known, Einthoven's is no less noteworthy.

Back to Mr. Valerian. What he suffered from is called Stokes-Adams Disease, a disorder resulting from a block in the conduction system between the atria and ventricles. This disease is complicated by episodes of unconsciousness which may or may not be associated with convulsions or seizures. Its recognition did not have to await the advent of clinical electrocardiography. In the *Dublin Quarterly Journal of Medicine* in 1846, Dr. William Stokes had provided the first complete clinical description of such a patient and remembered in his report the mention of another case twenty years earlier by a fellow Dubliner, Dr. Robert Adams.[7] What distinguished these cases of apoplexy (i.e., stroke) from other cases in which brain hemorrhage or clots could be demonstrated at autopsy was that they were associated with a perceptible marked slowing of the pulse. Furthermore, after each attack, with the exception of the final one, no paralysis of the limbs or other bodily motor functions resulted. The seat of the disorder was clearly in the heart and not the brain, but for another hundred years and more there was nothing definitive that physicians could do to treat it.

In the late 1940s, Dr. Paul M. Zoll was busy picking up his career in Boston after his military service in World War II.[8] He had followed the route of many clinical investigators within the Harvard system, combining private practice with hospital-based research. He was working under the eminent Dr. Herrman L. Blumgart, director of medical research at Beth Israel Hospital, and his close collaborator, the equally renowned pathologist Monroe J. Schlesinger. They were involved in a monumental study in which the hearts of more than twelve hundred consecutive autopsied patients were examined by coronary injection techniques and microscopic tissue analysis to determine correlations between the clinical and pathological findings in coronary heart disease.

A patient who came to Zoll in the late 1940s deflected his preoccupation with this work toward another direction. A "very nice lady," sixty years of age, suddenly had developed complete heart block with seizures typical of Stokes-Adams disease. The symptoms progressed rapidly, and within three weeks she was dead. At postmortem nothing other than disease of the conduction tissue was found, and Zoll was beside himself. "It was so damned frustrating. . . . It just wasn't right that she should die under our hands when nothing else was wrong with her."

Zoll had sought the advice of Blumgart and other experts, but they had had nothing to offer. He recalled the war years, working with his classmate, the surgeon Dwight Harken, who had removed shell fragments from the chests of wounded servicemen in England. He remembered how sensitive the hearts had been to mechanical stimuli, jumping with extra beats as they were manipulated intraoperatively. He also remembered how close the esophagus was to the heart, running right behind it through the chest down to the stomach. Surely there must be some practical way of stimulating the heart electrically to maintain an adequate rate, he thought.

He began to search the literature for clues to a solution and found that, in 1932, a prominent Brooklyn cardiologist, Albert B. Hyman, had been equally dismayed by physicians' inability to stimulate what he called "the stopped heart."

He had been moved to write, "In the brief interval before complete surrender to death has taken place, and before utter helplessness has seized those administering to the dying person, many random and badly executed procedures are invoked with the last minute hope of resuscitating the stopped heart."[9]

Zoll recognized that it was not the problem of Stokes-Adams disease that Hyman had addressed but the final culmination of cardiac disease in his patients. However, Hyman had been correct in emphasizing the futility of injecting cardiac stimulants willy nilly by inserting needles through the chest walls of dying patients, a procedure that had been in vogue since 1921. Hyman had pointed out that such drugs could, in excessive doses, be toxic instead of therapeutic. He had also raised the possibility that when heartbeats *were* induced, it might have been because of the stimulation by the needles rather than because of the medications.

In the laboratory Hyman had passed an electric current down a needle through the chest walls of laboratory animals to stimulate the right atrium in an attempt to mimic the normal course of cardiac conduction.[10] Zoll knew that in complete heart block he would have to stimulate the ventricles directly and that, although Hyman had mentioned some success in treating cardiac arrest in humans, he had never documented this by publication.

Zoll received additional encouragement in this pursuit following his attendance at a meeting of the Boston Surgical Society in 1950. Two Toronto surgeons, W. G. Bigelow and J. C. Callaghan, had been attempting experimental open-heart surgery by use of hypothermia—the lowering of the animal's body temperature so that the low metabolic activity of the heart thus induced would protect it from damage during temporary interruption of its blood supply. Excessive slowing or complete cessation of the heartbeat was a common accompaniment to these procedures, and at the Boston meeting Callaghan described how they had passed a wire electrode down to the heart via a jugular vein in these dogs so as to stimulate the heart in the region of the sinus node.[11]

Following the meeting, an excited Zoll questioned Callaghan and learned that the surgeons had simply been using a type of electrical stimulation that physiologists and pharmacologists had employed for years in animal experiments. The instrument in common use was a stimulator which could be obtained from the Grass Instrument Company, located in Quincy, Massachusetts. The key to a solution had been right next door to Boston all the time. Zoll approached the head of the Pharmacology Department at Harvard and "permanently borrowed" a unit that he used in his subsequent experiments.

In anesthetized dogs, he initially introduced one electrode down the esophagus, locating it right behind the heart, with another on the chest wall and a third for grounding elsewhere on the body. He first determined that extra beats could be induced in this way, and then, in anticipation of human application where time considerations would not permit esophageal insertion, he found that *both* stimulating electrodes could be placed externally, one on each side of the chest. Extensive studies were then undertaken to select proper strength, duration of electric charges, and so forth. Zoll was ready for his first human trial, which took place in the summer of 1952.

It was accepted that the first patient would have to be one so near death that the risk of electrocution or other harm was far outweighed by the natural course of the disease. The first candidate, a man in his eighties and the father of one of Zoll's neighbors, had been rushed to the emergency room of Beth

Israel Hospital in a terminal state. Zoll managed to pace him successfully for twenty minutes before he succumbed, but it was not from the pacing. There had been so many needles stuck through the chest wall to administer cardiac stimulants that one of these had nicked a cardiac vein. Blood from the vein had seeped into the pericardial sac surrounding the heart, and the patient died from cardiac tamponade.

A month later, a second patient was presented to Zoll at Beth Israel and was successfully paced for forty-eight hours. He was gradually weaned from the pacemaker and sent home on cardiac medications. Although the patient died six months later from another Stokes-Adams attack, Zoll felt confident that "we were on our way."[12]

As the work progressed, as with many new medical advances, the public and professional response was mixed. Along with the accolades came questions of morality posed by ethicists, self-appointed and otherwise. Was it really right to be interfering with divine will in such cases? Zoll took comfort from the support of his closest associates. Blumgart in particular was a tower of strength. But support could even come from unexpected sources. A monsignor, writing in the Catholic periodical, *The Pilot,* pointed out that God worked in many wondrous ways and that perhaps this cardiologist was one of His instruments. It amused Zoll to learn that a diminutive, rather reserved physician working at a Jewish hospital in Boston had been so designated.

In purely scientific terms, however, Zoll recognized that in a sense there were as many problems created as had been solved. To succeed in treating heart block patients, the pacemaker had to be in place and ready to go into action almost immediately. The brain cannot recover from a cessation of its blood supply that persists any longer than three or four minutes. Hospital organization and logistics of the time were unprepared for such an innovation.

At first, in patients with heart block, between Stokes-Adams attacks the electrodes were kept in place with a nurse in constant attendance. Immediately upon recognition of a dangerous slowing or arrest of heart rate, the nurse could activate the system. But this arrangement was inefficient and often ineffective. Inevitably, it seemed, the nurse would go to the bathroom or leave the bedside momentarily for some other reason, and precisely at that juncture the patient would convulse or die. "It was almost as if Stokes-Adams disease was a malignant intelligent being. Attacks would always happen at the worst possible time," Zoll recalls.

The solution was an electronic monitor that could sense the presence of electrocardiographic deflections and be set for automatic activation of the pacemaker whenever the heart rate fell below a predetermined rate. Zoll turned to Electrodyne, the firm with which he had associated himself, to build for him the prototype of all the cardiac monitors we see today in operating rooms, critical care units, and the like.

Like Hyman, Zoll realized that in the past cardiac stimulants had been injudiciously administered to patients with heart block. With a pacemaker at hand to maintain the heartbeat, a more rational approach to graded, physiological doses of such drugs could be developed. This technique was worked out with his associate, Dr. Arthur Linenthal. Instead of frantic intracardiac injections of concentrated cardiac stimulants, the drugs were diluted in saline or glucose solutions and titrated in drops-per-minute dosages to achieve the desired effect without inducing arrhythmias or other complications.[13]

Following the initial successes with Zoll's external pacemaker, modifications and improvements followed. Although not a problem in Zoll's first long-term survivor, chest pain resulting from chest muscle contraction and skin burns proved a formidable problem in many subsequent patients. It was this difficulty that led Furman and Uhley to explore the use of smaller currents with the use of transvenous intracardiac pacemakers. These were practical for temporary pacemaking in the presence of transitory heart block. In patients with permanent heart block, the presence of catheters emerging from the skin provided a convenient portal for infection. The solution was to internalize the entire system.

Following the lead of a Swedish surgical resident, Åke Senning, who demonstrated that a wire could be sutured to the heart and then attached to a portable power pack with the latter completely internalized under the skin,[14] a Buffalo surgeon, Dr. William M. Chardack, with Dr. Andrew A. Gage and engineer Wilson Greatbatch, popularized the "transistorized self-contained implantable pacemaker for the long term correction of complete heart block."[15] Initially, the wires were sutured directly to the exposed heart during thoracotomy; later, the transvenous technique was used to introduce the wire, eliminating the need for major chest surgery.

Construction of the early wires made them susceptible to early breakage. This was solved with the use of newly developed alloys. Electrode tips became increasingly ineffective because of foreign body reaction around them. This growth of tissue around the wire required periodic increases in current amplitude until replacement was mandatory. This difficulty was remedied by meticulous cleaning of the metallic surfaces, smoothing them to microscopic perfection. The earliest power packs, using mercury zinc oxide batteries, lasted only one to two years at most. The use of lithium-powered batteries has extended their life to approximately ten years. In certain cases of congenital heart block or that otherwise occurring in very young patients, nuclear-powered pacemakers with a shelf life of twenty years or more are now available.

It was soon found that the application of electric shocks to the chest wall was not only effective in heart block, but also useful in terminating a variety of rapid heartbeats originating either in the atria or in the ventricles. Perhaps most important was the use of this technique in the most serious and common electrical malfunction of all, sudden cardiac arrest resulting from coronary heart disease.

In 1926, officials at Consolidated Edison in New York City had become increasingly alarmed at the number of deaths of their linemen, killed by accidental electrocution. At the time there was no known method of reviving them. On the advice of a committee of experts at the Rockefeller Foundation, they decided to put some specialists at Johns Hopkins University to work on the problem. One was a neurologist, O. R. Langworthy; another, Professor R. D. Hooker, was a physiologist; and the third, William B. Kouwenhoven, was a professor of electrical engineering.[16]

Beginning in 1928, they made little progress until they were pointed in the right direction at a meeting called in 1930 by Dr. William H. Howell, chairman of the physiology department. Howell handed them a copy of a paper published in 1900 that he had come across. Two investigators at the University of Geneva, J. L. Prevost and F. Batelli, had reported that ventricular fibrillation, a lethal irregularity of cardiac rhythm, could be reversed in the open-chest dog heart by either alternating or direct current discharges.[17] (Incidentally, it would later be rediscovered that in 1775, 124 years before Prevost and Batelli, a remarkable Danish physician-veterinarian, Peter Christian Abildgaard, had reported essentially the same findings in a variety of animals to the Medical Society in Copenhagen.[18])

What Howell wanted to know was "Is it true?" and the Hopkins trio set out to answer this question to their own satisfaction in a series of investigations extending over two decades.

While the Hopkins group was still in the early stages of its work and had not yet reached the point of human application, Zoll, following the success he had already had with Stokes-Adams disease and other causes of cardiac standstill, soon realized that a major application for his device might be in acute myocardial infarction (heart muscle damage caused by severe coronary obstruction related to atherosclerotic narrowings, thrombi ("clots"), but usually a combination of both).

Of the 30 percent of patients with acute myocardial infarction dying in hospital, in about half of these the cause of death was an electrical failure of the heart. In some cases there would be complete cardiac standstill, but in the majority this would be preceded by failure of normal, coordinated contraction of the ventricles, which effectively reduced the pumping action of the heart to nil. The gross appearance of this problem was a heart that looked like a bundle of worms, with random, useless twitching of the many muscle bundles comprising the ventricles—ventricular fibrillation.

Zoll had been aware of important animal work that had been done with fibrillation-defibrillation in the 1940s at Cleveland's Western Reserve by a pioneer in cardiovascular physiology, Carl Wiggers, and his associates. Their studies were all in open-chest preparations, with the electrodes applied directly to the surface of the heart. In 1946 two Russian investigators, N. L. Gurvich and G. S. Yuniev, had demonstrated the feasibility of external defibrillation in dogs.[19] Zoll asked his engineer at Electrodyne, Alan Belgard, to build him a unit with externally applied paddles that would be effective in humans.

Another important later stimulus to Zoll's work also came from Western Reserve, this time in the person of an archetypically aggressive surgeon, Claude S. Beck. A pioneer cardiac and chest surgeon (see the chapter "Into the Heart"), Beck was well aware of the hazard of ventricular fibrillation in the operating room, where injudicious manipulation of the heart, anesthetics, lack of oxygen, or other poorly understood metabolic factors might lead to this fatal complication. In 1947, while closing the chest incision in a fourteen-year-old boy on whom he had operated for a severe funnel chest deformity, Beck found that the heart had suddenly arrested in ventricular fibrillation. The surgeon reopened the chest and, with the use of drugs and a defibrillator, was able to restore normal rhythm in the boy, who had been "apparently dead." The patient left the hospital without any ill effects from the episode.[20]

What kept the patient alive until the paddles of the defibrillator (obtained originally from Wiggers' laboratory) could be applied was Beck's enclosing the heart in his hands and substituting for the pumping action of the ventricles by squeezing ("massaging") it rhythmically until normal function could be restored.

In another dramatic episode, Beck was in the radiology department reviewing some films when a physician standing next to him collapsed in cardiac arrest. Beck immediately cut the chest open and massaged the heart until the patient could be resuscitated by the defibrillator.

What was emphasized by such cases as these was that manual compression of the exposed heart could temporarily replace the contraction of heart muscle until defibrillation could be accomplished. At the time closed-chest cardiac compression in humans was not established as a possible alternative. It would not be shown until the early 1960s that this could also substitute for the heartbeat.

In the early enthusiasm for open-chest cardiac resuscitation, the maintenance of proper ventilation was frequently overlooked or difficult to accomplish outside the surgical suite. Later infection could also be a problem, but perhaps the most feared event related to the fact that it was not always easy to be sure that cardiac arrest was the cause of some patient's seemingly unconscious appearance. Furthermore, no surgical resident was considered to be in proper uniform without a knife dangling from his key chain. In the gallows humor typical of the hospital corridor, we were all warned to beware of dozing off in the presence of some overzealous surgical acolyte. One could have one's chest cut open in the middle of an innocent snore under the prevailing attitude, which was only aggravated by the knowledge that the brain could not survive a lack of its blood supply for more than three or four minutes and *immediate* action was the only recourse.

In 1956, Zoll and his associates reported the first cases of successful cardiac resuscitation from ventricular fibrillation by external defibrillation in humans.[21] Similar reports soon emanated from Johns Hopkins, where in 1960 the effectiveness of *closed-chest* cardiac massage was also demonstrated. The noninvasive techniques of closed-chest cardiac massage, mouth-to-mouth respiration, and external defibrillation have all come together in what we all now recognize as CPR (cardiopulmonary resuscitation).

What about "cardiac arrest" outside the operating room, more specifically in patients with acute myocardial infarction? At postmortem examination, many of the patients succumbing to ventricular fibrillation were found to have only small amounts of heart muscle damaged by the incident of coronary occlusion. What had killed them was a "short circuit" set up in perhaps only a minute portion of the heart muscle, disrupting the normal cardiac rhythm and resulting in fibrillation. In the colorful phraseology introduced by Beck, "These were hearts too good to die."

In the late 1950s, a Kansas internist returning from a European trip, stopped by in Boston to visit Zoll. Dr. Hughes Day recognized the potential of constant monitoring with pacing or defibrillation when necessary in acute myocardial infarction and other serious cardiac ailments and saw the logistical problems that were plaguing Zoll. "Why don't you just build a special unit where you can put all these patients with the proper equipment and the proper personnel who know how to use it?" he asked. Zoll had found it impossible to institute such a setup at Beth Israel but gave Day his blessing to try it on his own when he got back to Kansas.

Day succeeded in funding a program for such a unit in Bethany, Kansas, and the CCU (Coronary Care Unit) was born. In short order Day clearly demonstrated the effectiveness of treating ventricular fibrillation and asystole (complete standstill) from myocardial infarction in such a setting.[22] The mortality from acute myocardial infarction dropped in half, from 30 to approximately 15 percent.

Progress in both permanent cardiac pacing and electrical termination of ventricular defibrillation has continued into the 1990s. For Zoll, the experience has come almost full circle thanks to a son who, at first, wanted nothing to do with medicine.

In 1969 the younger Zoll was about to finish undergraduate work at Harvard, and Blumgart, then serving as chairman of the medical school admissions committee and noting his excellent academic performance, asked Paul Zoll why the boy had not yet applied to the medical school. Blumgart was tentatively informed that Zoll's son was not sure he wanted to study medicine.

"Tell him to come see me." the great man confidentally advised the father. Some time later an amused Blumgart called Zoll again.

"Do you know what *your son* said to me? He said he would rather be a physicist if he can be a *good* physicist. If not, he would *consider* studying medicine!"

Ross Zoll went to Chicago and did become a good physicist but returned to Boston in 1976 and began working with his father. He was able to demonstrate that, with proper modifications, externally applied electrodes could be used for pacing without any painful muscle twitching or skin irritation. The current model can be quickly and easily applied, avoiding the risks and delay involved with inserting even a temporary pacing catheter.

Other improvements in pacemaking include the ability to reprogram permanent pacemakers in terms of rate, output, or other parameters simply by applying a device to the chest wall for a moment or two. In certain patients sequential pacing, that is, pacing first the atrium and then the ventricle using two different electrodes, can now be done. Newer devices in the process of development will enable the pacing rate to be change automatically through responses to body temperature, blood acidity, or muscular activity. Thus the natural changes in heart rate relative to variation in physical activity can be achieved.

A major new advance in defibrillation has also been introduced. Not all sudden deaths occur in the Coronary Care Unit. Many patients outside the hospital experience sudden death from ventricular fibrillation either as their first episode of coronary heart disease or as the late result of a previous myocardial infarction. After resuscitation, it can be predicted by electrophysiological studies which of these patients might be at a high risk for experiencing a second episode, one that might occur in the absence of any readily available life support personnel. Now, thanks to Dr. Michel Mirowski at Mt. Sinai Hospital and Johns Hopkins Medical School in Baltimore, an automatic implantable cardiac defibrillator has been developed.[23] The power pack is inserted under the skin, with the leads attached directly to the heart through chest surgery. The arrangement is reminiscent of that used for the early Chardack pacing device. Should an episode of fibrillation occur out of the hospital, the automatic defibrillator can sense the event and provide an internal shock to reverse it.

Much is currently being written about the tyranny of medical technology and how so many patients, indubitably contrary to their will if it could be expressed, are being artificially maintained in a vegetative state at great financial and emotional cost to their families and friends—perhaps their physicians as well. No doubt abuses exist and should be corrected. But for those of us who practiced medicine before the advent of such incredibly useful devices, the gains have far outstripped the disadvantages.

It has been said that each of us must struggle with the demons within. Certainly every physician is haunted by the spirits of patients past. For Zoll, it was that "nice lady" who was beyond his help. Herman Uhley will never forget Mr. Valerian. Mirowski was motivated to develop his automatic defibrillator by the devastating loss of a respected former chief and mentor to sudden cardiac death from a ventricular arrhythmia.

For this writer, there is not only the vivid recollection of Mr. Valerian. There was also a fading beauty in her early sixties who had suffered a massive myocardial infarction and whom I had befriended. Each night after finishing my intern's duties I would come to her bedside for a chat. I would hold her hand as we conversed and, almost unconsciously, maintain one finger on her pulse. One evening, in the midst of some story she was gaily recounting to me, I suddenly noticed that the pulse had stopped. Transfixed, I sat there helplessly while she calmly continued talking for a few more seconds before quietly slipping away.

But only three years or so after Mr. Valerian, there was Mr. Garibaldi, who was rushed to me following his first fainting attack from heart block in the spring of his eighty-ninth year. He had recovered consciousness by the time he had reached the hospital but was still in heart block with a dangerously slow rate.

Although there was some concern about how he would tolerate treatment at such an advanced age, a temporary pacemaker was introduced via a neck vein and later replaced with a permanent implantable device. Both procedures were performed without general anesthesia and with the patient fully awake. No complications of any kind occurred.

As Mr. Garibaldi was wheeled out of the heart cathetariza-tion laboratory after the permanent catheter and power pack had been put in place, he asked, "Hey Doc, how long do you think this thing is going to last?" When told that its life was two or possibly three years at most, he responded, "You mean I have to come back in two years for *another* one?"

To everyone's amazement but, possibly, his own, at the age of ninety-one he did indeed return for a replacement; then again at ninety-three and again at ninety-five. He died at the age of ninety-seven from noncardiac causes.

They all had "hearts too good to die."

Polio

The Not-So-Twentieth-Century Disease

On December 20, 1979, a historic decision was taken by the state of Georgia. The Board of Human Resources voted to permanently close the Warm Springs Hospital, where thousands of polio victims had received treatment, most prominently the first and most eminent, Franklin Delano Roosevelt. The future thirty-second president of the United States had been stricken with the disease in 1921 at the age of thirty-nine.

In 1924, still suffering from the paralysis which he would endure for the rest of his life, Roosevelt visited this rundown resort owned by a banker friend. He then first experienced the soothing and revivifying effects of the natural warm springs that gave the place its name. Roosevelt spent a good part of his paternal inheritance to purchase the property in 1926 and to rebuild and staff it in subsequent years. Warm Springs soon became a symbol of attempts to overcome the crippling effects of paralytic poliomyelitis.

The closing of Warm Springs evoked a note of sadness among those who had invested so much of their lives in its development. But, more important, it represented a moment of triumph. Polio had finally been eliminated as a major threat to the health of the nation. Perhaps no other disease—at least no viral disease—had so prominently endangered modern American society. No one, even today, who grew up in the 1940s or 1950s or before can forget the fear that each new summer brought with the menace of still another polio epidemic.

And yet, despite its impact on modern Western societies, so acutely recognized in the twentieth century—a time during which there was a flowering of medical knowledge and control of infectious diseases—during much of this period polio, like Churchill's Russia, remained "a riddle wrapped in a mystery inside an enigma."

The problems confronting investigators bent on eradicating polio were made all the more formidable by basic beliefs about it that persisted for generations, hampering progress against it. For example:

- It affected primarily the populations of modern, Western-type societies. *Wrong.*
- It was, by its nature, a children's disease. *Wrong.*
- It was caused by a single type of infectious agent. *Wrong.*
- It usually resulted in paralysis. *Wrong.*
- It attacked a person through the nose, working its way into the central nervous system via the peripheral nerve fibers ending there. *Wrong.*

Medical historians, searching back into antiquity, have found graphic evidence of lame children with the typical appearance of paralytic polio, suggesting that the disease has long been with us. It was not until the nineteenth century, however, that clinical descriptions of what we recognize as paralytic polio began to be undertaken. These more recent reports indicated for the first time that paralysis may not always result from a polio attack and that inapparent infections without subsequent paralysis might even constitute the majority among susceptible populations. Concurrently, neuropathologists, primarily in France, demonstrated the characteristic spinal cord lesions: destruction of the anterior horn cells of the cord, those responsible for motor function. Conversely, the sparing of sensory function was soon recognized as a hallmark of the disease. But what was the cause?[1]

Today we routinely accept the existence and nature of viruses for what they are, replicating tiny particles of nature that require living cells upon which to feed for their survival. But at the beginning of this century people argued as to whether or not they were simply small bacteria and whether or not they were living things at all. The triumphs of bacteriology, brought about over the past hundred years, can in great part be ascribed to the light microscope under which these larger microbes were revealed. But viruses were "invisible" until the invention of the electron microscope in the 1930s. Before that time the term "filterable viruses" *(virus* is Latin for "poison") was in vogue because, to isolate them, solutions were passed through porcelain filters with orifices small enough to prevent any bacteria from passing through but which would allow smaller particles to be recovered in the filtrate.

When asked how one studied viruses in 1923, for example, the colorful and curmudgeonly Dr. Thomas M. Rivers replied in later years "I think it's kind of a crime for a sinner like me to quote the Bible but . . . you shall know them by their deeds." In other words, you filtered them out, injected them into laboratory animals, and observed the effects.

Rivers was the rough-edged Georgia boy who entered the Rockefeller Institute in 1922 and remained there to become dean of American virologists until his retirement in 1955. Although not directly involved in a major part of laboratory research involving polio, he served as chief medical advisor of the National Foundation for Infantile Paralysis (NFIP) from 1955 until his death in 1962. As such, he profoundly influenced the thinking and direction of polio research throughout his active career.[2]

His routine at the Rockefeller might well have served as a model for all in pursuit of the elusive polio virus. He worked seven days a week from early morning until often after ten in the evening. As for the overstated role of serendipity in science, he observed, "I will admit that some great discoveries have been stumbled on by accident but, remember, you don't stumble unless you are walking. . . . There is no substitute for work in science."

Another workaholic, Dr. Karl Landsteiner (1868–1943) is

credited with first demonstrating the infectious nature of polio while still a young man in Vienna. He and his associate, Emil Popper, had taken the spinal cord of a boy who had died after a three-day illness and in whom cultures of the spinal cord were negative for bacterial growth. They injected the ground-up material into the abdominal cavity of two monkeys, one of whom died a week later; in the other a flaccid paralysis of the legs developed seventeen days later. At postmortem the spinal cords of both monkeys demonstrated anterior horn lesions strikingly similar to those described in human polio.

By 1909, Landsteiner and Popper, among others, had extended these observations, demonstrating that the infection could be passed from monkey to monkey. The viral etiology of polio became established beyond any doubt among the microbiological research community. Although Lansteiner joined the Rockefeller staff, he would not continue his work in polio. Among other interests, he was absorbed with blood typing in which he would perform pioneering work ultimately recognized with the awarding of a Nobel prize in medicine.

It was at the Rockefeller, however, that a major effort regarding polio was to be undertaken under its first director, Dr. Simon Flexner, a pathologist who had assumed this post only five years before Landsteiner's discovery and was among those who had successfully accomplished transmittal of polio among monkeys.[3] Despite his penetrating intelligence and impeccable scientific credentials, Flexner was responsible for perpetuating some major misconceptions about polio by failing to make distinctions between the disease he, as a basic scientist, studied in laboratory animals, and the human disease encountered in the field by practicing physicians. Flexner performed all of his studies in monkeys in which he believed that the virus was naturally transmitted only through the nasal passages where it infected the olfactory nerve fibers, involved the olfactory bulb at the base of the brain where these terminated and then finally spread to the spinal cord. Indeed, his monkeys were often infected by the rubbing of swabs dipped in virus-containing material against the mucous membranes in their noses.

So convincing was this belief about the transmission of polio

and so influential was Flexner and the Rockefeller Institute
among the medical community that, following the laboratory
demonstration that monkeys might be protected against polio
infection by intranasal sprays with certain irritating chemical
agents, human trials were soon undertaken. In Alabama, cor-
rosive substances such as picric acid and alum were sprayed
into the nasal passages of young children in order to protect
them against polio. The trial was a failure, and some of these
children lost their ability to smell for the rest of their lives.
After much discussion, many blind alleys, and despite the
nearly irresistible current of the Flexner dogma, it would
eventually be shown that the pathogenesis of polio in humans
involved the oral ingestion of virus, replication in the intestine, appearance in the bloodstream, and then final involvement of the central nervous system. It is currently believed
that this oral-fecal person-to-person spread is especially facili-
tated among playmates and family members sharing bathing
and toilet facilities.

Another source of confusion for early investigators was the
lack of recognition that there was more than a single type of
polio virus. Flexner, for most of his investigative career, maintained that there was only one type. It was not until 1949 that
Dr. David Bodian and his associates at Johns Hopkins University would unequivocally confirm what they and others had
previously suspected: there were actually three immunologically distinct types of polio virus. The development of a successful vaccine would require the inclusion of all three types in
order to succeed worldwide.

It also became important to recognize the significance of
"strain" versus "type" of polio. Each type represented a genetically distinct form of the virus so that antibodies produced in
response to one type would protect for that type only and not
the other two. Within each type, however, there could be
dozens of strains, all linked immunologically because of a similar genetic structure, but capable of varying markedly in their
clinical manifestations: infectivity, growth characteristics, virulence, and so on. Sometimes the names given to these strains
related to the locale in which they were isolated (for example,

the Lansing strain) or a patient in whom one was found (for example, the Mahoney strain). Occasionally such designations could be rather fanciful, the Brunhilde strain, for example, being named for a chimpanzee whose physical and personal attributes suggested the title.

At the Rockefeller, the selection of the so-called MV strain was convenient in that it reproducibly caused the death of monkeys following paralysis of all four limbs when injected into their brains. Unfortunately though, through repeated passages in laboratory animals, it had become highly neurotropic (that is, infecting only nervous tissue), whereas natural-occurring polio would be shown to infect a number of tissues. The specificity of this strain for nervous tissue would lead to confusion and failure when later attempts were made to culture polio virus on nonnervous tissue using only the MV strain.

Although a brief summary such as this must, of necessity, omit mention of a number of individuals whose contributions were of great value, no reference to polio could possibly be made without the inclusion of Dr. Albert B. Sabin's remarkable accomplishments.[4] From 1931, when his interest in the disease began during an epidemic in New York City, to the present, his personal history has been inextricably entwined with the disease for which his vaccine was developed. In his youth and middle years, his photographs presented a dapper, even dandified figure with prematurely gray hair and an almost pencil-thin Hollywood moustache. They belied the true character of this tireless, painstaking investigator with a ferocious desire to seek out the truth even when it overturned his own previous conceptions and experimental data. Now a portly, fully bearded patriarch in his ninth decade, he retains an encyclopedic grasp of the past events surrounding the polio story and a continuing interest in spreading the benefits of modern preventive medicine throughout the less fortunate countries of the third world.

An immigrant from Bialystok in Russo-Poland who arrived in the United States at the age of fifteen, Sabin showed research promise at an early age after switching from the study of dentistry to medicine. Following his graduation from New York University's Medical School, his formal training and work in infectious disease began in the Department of Bacteriology at NYU and the Lister Institute in London. He then worked at the Rockefeller Institute from 1935 to 1945 before moving to the Children's Hospital Research Foundation at the University of Cincinnati Medical School.

Perhaps Dr. Sabin's tenacity in approaching a research problem can best be exemplified by an early episode in his career, one that only peripherally involved the polio virus. After being hired as a research assistant by Dr. William H. Park at NYU, he was assigned to work on polio. Later there was another newcomer to the department, a young Canadian, Dr. William Brebner. In the course of their work, Brebner was bitten by a monkey. He soon after developed paralysis which progressively and fatally involved his respiratory center and other parts of the brain. Sabin examined a number of tissues obtained from the autopsy and reported that he had discovered a new virus, one he intended to call the Brebner virus after his unfortunate coworker. (The name was later changed to "B virus" by the ultraproper editor of the *Journal of Experimental Medicine*, Dr. Peyton Rous.[5])

The professor and head of the bacteriology department at Columbia University's College of Physicians and Surgeons at the time was Dr. Frederick Gay, a recognized world authority on herpes-type viruses. He had also acquired autopsy material from the Brebner postmorten and declared that the virus involved was simply one of the herpes type. The very junior (at the time) Sabin refused to give ground and received support from Tom Rivers to whom he showed his work. He then proceeded to test other monkeys in New York looking for the B virus but with no success. When he went to work at the Lister Institute, he again sought the virus in laboratory monkeys and this time was able to obtain confirmation of his earlier finding concerning Brebner's death. Some years later, in Cincinnati, he received a call in the middle of the night from a pathologist who had recalled Sabin's paper just as he was about to perform an autopsy on a pharmacologist whose job had been to feed laboratory monkeys various test preparations. Just prior to his paralytic fatal illness, the pharmacologist had cut his finger with a tin vial cap and then accidentally contaminated the small wound with saliva from one of the monkeys in his charge. His autopsy was presided over by Sabin, and again the B virus was found. Sabin continued to collect cases, confirming and reconfirming the work with the deaths of other laboratory workers and even a member of the royal Greek family who died after receiving a monkey bite.

Today the B virus is recognized as a common infection in monkeys where it is seldom of major consequence although nearly always fatal when transmitted to humans.

Sabin has proved just as unrelenting in testing the validity of his own polio work and that of his closest associates. While at the Rockefeller Institute under Flexner, he was the first to demonstrate pathologically under the microscope the olfactory bulb lesions produced in monkeys by swabbing their nasal passages with virus.

By the time he arrived in Cincinnati, Sabin felt compelled to pursue this further. From colleagues in Chicago, where an epidemic was raging, he obtained olfactory bulbs from human autopsies in fatalities that had occurred. The human olfactory bulbs were perfectly normal. Obviously there was something radically different in the transmission of human polio and experimental polio observed in the Rockefeller's laboratory monkeys.

In Cincinnati, Sabin and his new young assistant, Robert Ward (See the chapter "Why Do They Turn Yellow?"), then collected tissues from various body sites in humans who had succumbed to polio. They demonstrated that the alimentary tract was consistently involved and probably an important site for viral replication.[6] This would be a key factor in the future selection of an oral type of vaccine that Sabin and his colleagues would prepare.

Like many great investigators, Sabin had the misfortune of devising an experiment, faultless in both design and execution, which only later would be shown to be dead wrong. While in Peter Olitsky's laboratory at the Rockefeller in 1936, he demonstrated for the first time that the polio virus could be cultivated *in vitro*, that is, in a culture of embryonic human tissue outside a living being. Unfortunately, it was the Rockefeller MV strain that was used in this study, and the only tissue on which the virus could be cultivated was neural in type. This perpetuated the false belief that the polio virus was exclusively neurotropic until, thirteen years later, Dr. John F. Enders and his associates, using the Lansing (Type II) strain, were able to culture the virus in embryonic cells of the intestine, liver, kidney, heart, and other tissues.[7] The tissue culture work of Enders and his coworkers, Drs. Thomas H. Weller and Frederick C. Robbins, was critical in the advancement of research in polio as well as other viral diseases. Prior to 1949, for the most part polio could only be studied by injecting the virus into susceptible monkeys and analyzing the pathological results. Now the virus could be studied "in the test tube," where Enders was able to detect what he called a "cytopathologic effect" on the cells under the microscope, a characteristic change in their appearance which resulted from viral multiplication.

Curiously enough, these tissue culture experiments were initially carried out primarily for the study of the mumps virus. As Enders remarked in his Nobel address, "close at hand in the storage cabinet was the Lansing strain of poliomyelitis virus. Thereupon it suddenly occurred to us that everything had been prepared almost without conscious effort on our part for a new attempt to culture the agent in extraneural tissue."

In the interim between the Sabin attempt to culture the virus in 1936 and Enders's work in 1949, a series of other revelations combined to bring polio research to the threshold of an effective vaccine.

Epidemiologic knowledge of the disease was an important component to this body of information. Once thought to be specifically a disease of childhood ("infantile paralysis"), polio, began to occur during World War II in outbreaks among Allied servicemen in far off parts of the world where previously it had been disregarded as a major problem. In Egypt, for example, an outbreak occurred in 1940–41 among British troops, all between twenty and forty years of age. Serological testing of the native population later revealed immunologic evidence of previously unexpected widespread prior exposure to the virus. Later, careful searches were made among such populations and evidence of previous paralytic polio, also not recognized before, turned out to be at least as common as in modern Western countries.

The reasons for the disparate patterns of polio in these different types of cultures became apparent. In Western societies, prior to the nineteenth and twentieth centuries when sanitary conditions became vastly improved, and in currently underdeveloped countries, newborns and infants became exposed to the virus very early in life. The virus was constantly present and widespread in such communities, but older groups, having been exposed in the past and having acquired immunity, for the most part were protected. In other words, polio was "endemic" in such environments. In the West, as more advanced hygienic conditions became standard, transmission of the virus in early life was less easily accomplished, and many individuals grew through childhood and into adulthood without previous exposure and without protective antibodies. When what the epidemiologists call a "critical mass" of susceptibles were present and virus was introduced and readily available for transmission (for example, during the summer months), the characteristic July and August epidemics were likely to occur. In this way, there arose the false impression of polio as a twentieth-century epidemic summer disease, occurring exclusively in advanced Western societies.

Extensive serological testing among populations exposed to the virus also made it clear that approximately 95 percent of all polio infections are subclinical, with no symptoms whatsoever. In 4 to 8 percent there may be fever, headaches, muscle pains, and so forth, typical of what we often recognize in many viral infections. Frank paralysis apparently occurs in only one of every thousand individuals infected with the polio virus.

In the laboratory, other advances were made helping facilitate the final attack on polio. In 1939, preceding Ender's work, Dr. Charles Armstrong of the Public Health Service was able to achieve infection of rats and then mice with a Lansing strain of polio. Before this, only monkeys and apes were found to be susceptible to the virus in the laboratory. Now that great numbers of expensive monkeys were no longer necessary, larger laboratories could effect economies, and smaller laboratories interested in studying aspects of the disease could now afford to get into the act, expanding the possibilities for new discoveries. A few years later, in 1946, Dr. Max Theiler at the Rockefeller showed that by serially passing Armstrong's Lansing virus through mice (fifty-two times in all), he was able to convert this pathologic strain to one that was harmless to susceptible monkeys. With 150 passages of the strain, it became not only harmless but capable of immunizing monkeys against future challenges with active Lansing Type II polio.

Whereas Theiler demonstrated that repeated passages of polio virus could induce mutations to attenuate the virus, Dr. Isabel Morgan at Johns Hopkins showed that by treating polio virus with formalin, it could not only be inactivated but also provide immunization in rhesus monkeys (that is, stimulate the production of antibodies). Thus, methodologies were now at hand for producing two types of polio vaccines, involving killed or live attenuated virus.

In addition, under the aegis of the NFIP, a massive effort was undertaken in 1948 to classify into the three recognized types of polio the 196 strains that had been independently studied and acquired from laboratories all over the world. This relatively dull but vitally important backbreaking effort to create order out of chaos was apportioned out to several laboratories in the United States, one of them at the University of Pittsburgh where Dr. Jonas Salk was at work.

Finally, by this time it was importantly recognized that viremia (presence of infective virus in the bloodstream) was involved in the pathogenesis of the disease and that the induction of circulating antibodies in the blood by a vaccine was the key to protection.

The stage seemed to be set for the proper vaccine. Certainly, other efforts to contain or treat the disease had not met with any huge success. Gamma globulin trials to protect children at risk had some value but were expensive and cumbersome. Furthermore, injection of this antibody-containing blood fraction collected from previously exposed volunteers with acquired immunity provided only temporary protection. Such injected antibodies did not stimulate antibody production by the recipient's own immune system, and, over time, they were gradually removed from the bloodstreams of those so treated. The following summer these children would be just as susceptible to infection as they had been prior to receiving gamma globulin a year before.

Much effort had been focused on rehabilitation of polio victims. The Warm Springs Hospital was more of a showplace than a major treatment center given its limited capacity, but did help in fund raising and served as an example to other therapeutic programs. Sister Kenny, a dedicated and driven Australian nurse, introduced a number of improvements in the acute and chronic management of paralyzed limbs. The NFIP, headed by FDR's former law partner, Basil O'Connor, continued to raise funds for research and public education. The annual March of Dimes campaign against polio with its posters of adorable children trapped in leg braces became an annual event in all our lives.

Strictly speaking, there was not much that one could do medically except to keep the acutely ill patient alive. A particularly ominous clinical type of polio was the "bulbar" type in which the motor cells higher up along the spinal cord and in the base of the brain were affected. This often resulted in weakness of paralysis of the muscles of the head, neck, and, most important, those responsible for respiration.

Invention of the so-called iron lung by Dr. Philip Drinker at the Harvard School of Public Health proved lifesaving in cases of respiratory failure, but even then the problems of medical management were incredibly complex. Boston's Dr. Louis Weinstein, an infectious disease specialist, once calculated that in his career he had treated about thirty-five hundred cases of polio during his years at various Boston Hospitals (more than one might now see in an entire lifetime throughout the United States, thanks to the polio vaccines). His recollections about

caring for patients in such respirators were graphic and rivet-
ing even thirty years later:

> I've always said that if one really wanted to find out how good
> an internist he was, he should take care of some patients with
> paralytic poliomyelitis. They had all kinds of problems. They
> had electrolyte and fluid problems. Because they were under
> such high stress, they had multiple stress ulcers from the
> fundus of the stomach right down to the rectum, so we had
> problems with gastrointestinal bleeding. I saw three or four pa-
> tients who, while very quietly lying in their respirators, rup-
> tured the esophagus and were found to have large stress ulcers
> postmortem. About a third, at least, of the adults had paralyzed
> bladders, so we got into all sorts of trouble with urinary tract
> infections and kidney stones. Since they were lying in respira-
> tors, and could not ventilate well, we saw pneumonias in large
> numbers. The psychiatric problems were innumerable, so that,
> in fact, we had an attending psychiatrist coming each day to
> visit the patients, especially during the 1955 epidemic.[8]

Because surgeons and obstetricians, for fear of transmitting
the disease to their other patients elsewhere, were reluctant to
attend polio patients at the Haynes Memorial, a communicable
disease hospital, Weinstein the internist was also obliged to de-
liver babies and perform appendectomies among other surgical procedures as the need arose. Most hair-raising, however,
was an experience with the respirators during that 1955 epidemic. Suddenly, one morning, with two dozen patients on
electrically powered units, the current failed and there was no
emergency backup generator available at the chronically
short-funded aging institution. Doctors, nurses, cooks, and
other hospital workers, garage mechanics, and firemen pulled
off the street were enlisted in the physically exhausting effort
to keep the respirators manually operated until power was restored nine hours later. Funds for the backup generator were
found soon thereafter.

The polio problem cried out for solutions, and by 1950, as
Dr. John R. Paul of Yale put it, the "decks (were) cleared for
action on a vaccine." Yet it was not without some feeling of
trepidation that the preeminent virologists of the time pre-

pared for such a step. Many of them had been present during the 1935 fiascos of two such attempts at a vaccine, both of which had resulted in failure and disgrace.

In the early thirties, presaging in some way the later rivalry between Salk and Sabin, two investigators emerged in competition with their respective polio vaccines. One, Dr. Maurice Brodie, had started in Montreal his studies with a formalin-inactivated (that is, dead) virus prepared from an emulsion of monkey spinal cord. Later, joining Sabin's first chief, Dr. Park, at the Department of Health in New York City, he embarked upon a human program in three thousand children after preliminary trials in only twenty monkeys. Their precipitous action was probably stimulated by the knowledge that Dr. John A. Kolmer in Philadelphia had developed a live attenuated vaccine, achieved, he claimed, by treatment of an active virus with sodium ricineolate, a soapy substance, combined with several other ingredients. In the summer of 1935, it was distributed throughout the country and administered to more than ten thousand children.

In both instances, the vaccines had been introduced prematurely. Knowledge about polio was still fragmentary in 1935: the three immunologic types had yet to be identified, for example. Animal and human trials had been totally inadequate. Protection by the vaccines used was questionable; what was not were the deaths of a number of children as a direct result of having been administered the vaccines. Both Brodie and Kolmer were publicly excoriated by their colleagues, the blunt Rivers prominently among them. Although Kolmer survived the episode professionally, Brodie, the prior recipient of so many attractive offers from so many outstanding laboratories, suddenly found himself a pariah. He finally accepted a minor position at an obscure midwestern institution and died soon after, allegedly by his own hand.

Fifteen years later, the options for a vaccine prepared with either a killed or live attenuated virus were still open, and both had precedents, advantages, and disadvantages.

Sabin and others opting for a live attenuated virus could point to previous successes with such vaccines. The prevention

of smallpox through use of the immunologically related cowpox by Jenner was the classic example. In more recent times,
Max Theiler at the Rockefeller Institute had developed precisely such a vaccine for yellow fever and won a Nobel prize in
medicine for it. But what proved the most convincing for
Sabin regarding the advantage of a live virus over a killed one
was its demonstrated long-lasting immunological protective effects. He had been greatly impressed by a 1949 study among
Eskimos by John Paul and his group. There had been an outbreak of polio in 1930 at a remote Alaskan village, with no
recurrences over the subsequent nineteen years. Serological
testing of more than two hundred inhabitants revealed that of
129 Eskimos under the age of twenty, there was complete absence of antibodies to Type II polio, whereas among those
over twenty years of age, 80 percent had antibodies to the virus. Protection acquired by exposure in 1930 had persisted for
twenty years.[9] For Types I and III infections, the case appeared the same.

The other option, the one eventually pursued by Jonas Salk,
was to use killed (inactivated) virus, which also had moderate
success in the control of another virus disease, influenza.

In 1951, in order to monitor and promote such efforts, the
NFIP, the primary funder of polio research at the time, set up
a Committee on Immunization, including among its membership the likes of Rivers, Enders, Paul, Bodian, Sabin, and a
relative newcomer to the polio scene, Dr. Jonas E. Salk.[10]

Salk, then thirty-seven years of age, is described at the time
by Paul as "a slight man who radiated a sort of restless eager-
ness and energy." A New Yorker who had graduated from
New York University's Medical School and spent five years
working under a prominent virologist, Dr. Thomas Francis,
Jr., at the University of Michigan. Salk then moved on to the
University of Pittsburgh, where his polio research was conducted.

Despite his relative youth, Salk had already by this time undergone experiences that would particularly suit his entry into
the field of polio vaccine development. Salk recalls how, as a
medical student in 1936, he attended two back-to-back lec-

tures in immunology that seemed to him to be totally incon-
sistent. In the first, the students were told that people could be
immunized against certain bacterial diseases (for example,
diphtheria and tetanus) by use of chemically treated toxins
from these microorganisms. In the following lecture, one concerning viruses, they were told that only with the use of a related live virus (as Edward Jenner had used cowpox against
smallpox) or an attenuated live virus (as Max Theiler had
done with yellow fever) could the immunological protective
response be produced. Salk had previously interrupted his
standard medical training for a year's study of biochemistry,
which had given him further insight into such problems.

His work with Francis culminated in the development of a
formalin-inactivated virus vaccine against influenza, the first
successful "killed vaccine" against a viral infection. Although
the emergence of various new strains of influenza virus would
confound later attempts to prevent or control future flu epidemics, the inclusion by Salk and Francis of a strain that was
to become prevalent at the time of their trial led to its effectiveness when applied in the large field trial of 1943.

This experience convinced Salk that so-called inactivated or
killed viruses would, in time, be the way to control or prevent
virus infections. The validity of this prediction, he maintains,
will be revealed in time, although the current "score" on this is
inconclusive. Bacterial diseases such as pertussis (whooping
cough) and cholera are controlled with killed vaccines, and
inactivated portions or products of microorganisms are effective in hepatitis B and diphtheria. On the other hand, live attenuated vaccines continue to be the preferable products used
in such widespread diseases as measles, mumps, and German
measles (rubella).

The opportunity to participate in the polio-typing effort
allowed Salk to familiarize himself with what was, for him, a
new organism. With the funds supplied for the typing program, he was also able to equip his new laboratory in Pittsburgh for future endeavors in viral research.

When it came to developing a vaccine to protect against
polio, the prior success with influenza, no doubt, was a strong

influence in tilting Salk toward a killed virus type of vaccine, as was the desire to avoid the risk of causing polio even with an attenuated virus vaccine. The problems confronting him in polio were still substantial. Not least among them was the need to master tissue culture techniques for the growing of all three types of polio virus with high antigenicity (ability to promote the production of antibodies). Also facing Salk and his associates was the need to determine precisely the right amounts of formalin treatments for each of the types. Too little might fail to inactivate the virus and thus result in causing infection and disease among recipients; too much might impair the antigenicity of the final preparation.

The problems facing Sabin were also formidable. Species differences encountered in response to polio virus were in themselves a plague to anyone pursuing this course of research. It was learned that as one progressed along the evolutionary ladder from monkey to humans, infection of the intestinal tract with virus became easier (that is, relatively difficult in the monkey, easier in chimpanzees, and easiest in humans). However, the propensity for nerve tissue damage after exposure to polio virus was exactly the opposite: virus strains that readily paralyzed monkeys were much less virulent to chimps and, presumably, humans. Complicating this set of circumstances regarding infectivity and virulence was the fact that these characteristics were independent of one another in the various known strains and could vary in opposite directions in any strain studied.

Thanks to previous work, much of it his own, Sabin knew that he would have to find viral strains that, as in naturally occurring human polio, would readily replicate in the intestine after oral administration. The major task was to find strains that would do that for all three polio types and yet not result in paralysis after administration.

As a result of Enders's great work, much of this testing could now be performed "in test tubes," but there was still one final problem for all those working to develop a live attenuated virus for a vaccine, their bête noire, in fact. There was always the possibility that after developing a harmless attenuated virus and administering it to a patient, they would find that in the process of multiplication within the gut, the virus would back-mutate to a virulent form which might cause clinical disease among contacts. This was more than just a theoretical possibility. Sabin himself had shown in monkey experiments that virus samples obtained from the stools of those who had received attenuated virus by mouth could become more virulent in character when they emerged and were fed to other laboratory animals.

Meanwhile, public pressure for a vaccine, transmitted through the directorship of the NFIP to its investigators, began to weigh more and more heavily upon all those concerned. When the Immunization Committee seemed incapable of moving ahead more decisively in its deliberations, the NFIP in 1953 appointed a new body, the Vaccine Advisory Committee, composed mainly of public health experts rather than laboratory researchers to "break the log jam," as one official put it.

As it turned out, by this time Salk and his associates had made more progress with the development of a killed virus vaccine than Sabin and others had made with an attenuated virus. By 1953, Salk had established the safety of his vaccine by a trial in patients previously paralyzed by polio, inmates of the Watson Home for Crippled Children in Leetsdale, Pennsylvania. This initial effort in humans was followed by others which demonstrated not only the safety of the vaccine, but its ability to stimulate the production of antibodies. By 1954, Salk had accumulated studies in nearly five thousand subjects, and the NFIP pushed even harder for a nationwide massive field trial. In 1954, just such an effort was made among nearly two million children in forty-four states.

Although marred subsequently by the "Cutter incident," in which some improperly prepared batches of vaccine had contained live virus and resulted in paralytic polio in several children, the trial had already demonstrated beyond doubt the effectiveness of the Salk-type vaccine.[11] It received governmental approval, and, with widespread administration in the United States between 1954 and 1961, the rate of paralytic

polio fell from 13.9 per 100,000 to 0.5 per 100,000, after a
peak of approximately 25 per 100,000 in 1953.

Despite the success of the 1954 trial, recollections of the
events leading up to it are tainted with some misgivings about
how the whole problem was handled, and the respective roles
of Salk and Sabin. For those with the narrow view that Salk
was rash and opportunistic in promoting his vaccine, it must
be noted that, preceding the 1954 trial, Rivers had described
Salk as overly cautious ("I can tell you that if I had a kid, I
wouldn't have hesitated for one minute to inoculate him at
that time [February 1953] with Salk's vaccine. Damn it, do you
know that at this meeting, Salk wouldn't even call his vaccine a
vaccine; he kept calling it an inactivated preparation.") For
those who believe that Sabin's only role was to undermine
Salk's efforts, it should be emphasized that he acknowledged
Salk's accomplishments but, along with Enders and others, felt
that live virus vaccine was the final way to go. In any event,
both were soon submerged in the train of events that took
place in the months preceding the trial. The future control of
polio was deemed too important to be in the hands of any one
laboratory or another. In the words of John Paul, the polio
program had essentially been "taken over" by the NFIP.

Meanwhile, development of an effective and live virus vaccine proceeded systematically and without fanfare in the laboratories of Sabin and others. Nevertheless, the success of the
Salk-type vaccine and the continuing fear that any live virus
might back-mutate after administration prompted some
prominent virologists to suggest that they desist. Sabin recalls
Rivers suggesting to him that he simply "throw my vaccine
into the nearest sewer." He chose not to.

Between 1954 and 1957, Sabin had achieved the selection of
the desired strains and tested them on monkeys, chimpanzees,
and more than one hundred human volunteers including his
own wife, two children, and several of their neighborhood
playmates, who were all found to be triple negative for the
three types of polio virus.

It should be noted at this point that self-experimentation in
vaccine development is often more the rule than the exception
as compared to other developments in medical science. Salk

also used himself and his family to test out his vaccine, as did others who worked along these lines. Although such practices might seem a bit startling, on further reflection their logic is undeniable. As the salty Rivers put it, "It's not that one expects to learn a lot by taking such material—one guy or his family proves nothing. But . . . I know that if anyone came up to me and asked me to take an untried vaccine I'd ask him 'Have you taken it?' and, by God, if that person said no I'd tell him to go to hell.")

Although the NFIP continued to give lip service to continued research on an oral live virus polio vaccine, in practical terms, what with the success of the Salk vaccine, attempts to promote it were essentially abandoned by the NFIP officialdom.

Virtually left in limbo by policymakers at home, Sabin and others working on the live vaccine later gained considerable international support from the World Health Organization at its 1957 conference on poliomyelitis. A strong recommendation was made for extensive trials of a live attenuated type of oral vaccine. This was welcome news not only to Sabin but to Drs. Hilary Koprowski and Harold Cox at Lederle Laboratories, who had been developing their own strains for an oral vaccine. However, since the latter later proved inadequately attenuated under the WHO guidelines, it was Sabin who ultimately "got the nod." Fortunately, having ignored Rivers's advice regarding sewerage disposal, Sabin recalls with relish, "I just happened to have twenty-five million doses of each of the important types ready for such trials."

The situation was not very propitious in the United States for an oral vaccine trial at the time. The Salk vaccine program was in full swing and effective there. Sabin turned to other more receptive areas—Czechoslovakia, Mexico, and especially the Soviet Union where by the end of 1959 about fifteen million people had received the oral vaccine and where the back-mutation bugaboo had failed to materialize.[12] The success of the Sabin vaccine abroad finally resulted in a rare endorsement by the American Medical Association. This was the opening wedge to its adoption in the United States.

Although the injectible Salk-type vaccine continued to be

used with great effectiveness in developed countries such as Sweden, Holland, and Finland where stringent schedules for vaccination could be enforced, in the United States since 1962 and in third world countries where governmental controls are less easily exerted, the Sabin oral vaccine has become the standard. Thus both types of vaccine have been shown to be effective, and if either type were the only one available, there would be no question about its efficacy and safety. Nevertheless, thanks to the longevity and determination of the principals, controversy over the relative advantages and disadvantages of the two types of vaccine continued to rage up to the present.

A detailed consideration of this issue is beyond the scope of this book and beyond the presumption of this reporter. But, in brief, what one wishes from an ideal vaccine is primarily only two things: that it be completely safe and completely effective. Arguments from one end of the spectrum and opinion about polio vaccination to the other continue to ping-pong back and forth down the years. They run (roughly!) something like this:

—Proponents of the killed vaccine can point to its undisputed safety record, especially in countries like Holland and Sweden where it has been used exclusively for years. Conversely, they point to the United States, where the live vaccine has been in use since 1962 and where approximately five to ten cases of vaccine-associated paralytic polio are still occurring each year. They contend that even one case of paralytic polio is too many if it can be prevented.

—Proponents of the live vaccine challenge the validity of the statistics from relatively homogeneous populations in Holland and Sweden as incomparable to those of the United States. They point to the ability of intestinal viruses other than polio to cause paralysis and do not consider the recovery of polio virus from the stools of such patients as incontrovertible proof that the polio virus was the culprit. They might also add that, whatever the risk of polio from live virus administration, the risk of the disease from ineffective killed virus among other populations might result in an equal or greater number of paralytic cases. They would emphasize that a major advantage of the live virus is its multiplication in the intestines of those to whom it is administered, with transmission of virus and protection to contacts who may not have even received any vaccine from health workers. Further in favor of the live attenuated virus would be its induction of intestinal immunity against any wild virus that might be subsequently introduced.

—The killed virus camp could counter with the improved antigenicity of more recent forms of this vaccine and thus its equal effectiveness to that of the live virus. They would pooh-pooh the importance of intestinal immunity: it is the immunity to paralysis that is important. They might be quick to point out that in terms of protection in tropical countries, for reasons poorly understood, the orally administered live virus is less effective than elsewhere.

—The live virus contingent can point to failures of the *killed* virus in certain tropical areas. The killed virus supporters point to failures of the live virus to protect the nonvaccinated even when very large numbers of other children have received the oral vaccine . . . and so on.

As late as 1987 two investigators at Johns Hopkins, Drs. A Marshall McBean and John F. Modlin, came up with a Solomonic proposal for immunization that might incorporate the best features and eliminate the deficiencies of both types of vaccine. They published a paper in which a regimen incorporating *both* types of vaccine might work out to the best advantage of the public.[13] Following this came two invited commentaries, one by Sabin and one by Salk, each eminently logical and reasonable by itself, each coming to a totally different conclusion regarding the exclusive use of either the oral live attenuated vaccine or the killed injectible preparation.

The future of polio immunization may well depend on legal considerations as well as scientific ones. An increasing number of litigations stemming from cases of paralysis related to oral live polio vaccine have begun to appear in the courts. In 1988 a Supreme Court ruling in such a case has made it likely that the federal government itself might become liable for damages in the event of negligence by its agents or agencies concerning "specific mandatory directives."

Be that as it may, current public policy recommends the

killed virus vaccine only in certain groups at increased risk
of paralytic polio as a result of the orally administered live
virus vaccine (for example, immunodeficient patients and
their families). For the majority, the oral polio vaccine is still
recommended. However, in 1987 the Public Health Service
requested the Institute of Medicine to grapple with this problem, and their 1988 report suggests that a combined approach
will most likely be the future plan. They recognized that, although an immediate switch to the enhanced killed vaccine
might eliminate the problem of vaccine-related paralytic polio,
it might also increase the incidence of wild virus infections
with paralytic disease. No doubt cognizant of the McBean/
Modlin rationale, the Institute's report looked forward to the
future incorporation of enhanced killed virus in the routine
DPT (diphtheria/pertussis/tetanus) injections during early infancy, with administration of the live oral polio vaccine at
eighteen months and upon entrance into elementary school.

As for the principal actors in this medical drama, in purely
philosophical terms perhaps Jonas Salk, himself, expresses
best the reason for their dichotomy of views:

> Different people have different perceptions; different people
> have different value systems; and the same things apply to sci-
> entists as they do to other human beings. You present me with
> a problem and I see it my way; you present someone else with a
> problem and he sees it his way. . . . Sabin is a virologist and I
> am an immunologist. Virologists don't trust the immune sys-
> tem; they trust the virus. I trust the immune system, not the
> virus. . . . In time, if we look at this from an evolutionary point
> of view we will see what will ultimately prevail.

Perhaps we should leave it at that and let the future determine scientific validity. Scientists, however, are just as fasci-
nated by controversy as anyone else, even more so when it
concerns their own world. Leaving out here the personal aspects of the polio vaccines' development would be like omit-
ting mention of the Red Sea in the retelling of the Exodus of
the Jews out of Egypt and into the promised land.

No doubt, at the time he emerged as a prominent figure in

polio research, Salk, then in his late thirties, was looked upon as something of a "whippersnapper" by those who had already dedicated much of their own professional lives to the problem and were still active in the field. Sabin, for all his great qualities ("my idea of a splendid man for research" according to Rivers), must have been particularly galling to Salk at times. According to Rivers, "Albert not only looked directly at the question, he looked around it, examined every possible facet, including a few theoretical facets that didn't occur to others."

Salk also did not appreciate Sabin's penchant for what some felt was sophisticated self-promotion. But if Sabin was accused of blowing his own horn on occasion, one had to admit that it was a horn of Wagnerian proportions. And he was not alone in his championing of an oral attenuated virus; he was joined by others, notably John Enders, Joseph Melnick, and Hilary Koprowski. They were all not simply bent on frustrating Salk's attempts at a vaccine. They all sincerely believed that there was a better way.

Sabin was also filled with resentment, in his case about the lukewarm response of the polio establishment to his efforts after the development of an oral attenuated viral vaccine that represented the culmination of more than twenty years of sustained intensive effort. Understandably, for their part, the controlling powers within the NFIP were gratified by the initial success of the Salk vaccine, and wanted time for long-term study of its effectiveness. Perhaps the last thing in the world they wanted at the time was another vaccine to test, even though it might have potential advantages over the Salk vaccine (as well as failings). Such considerations, however, were small comfort to Sabin, and one can well imagine how all of Sabin's frustrations of this period might have been embodied in the person of the man whose killed vaccine was blocking the introduction of his own dearly won and highly prized innovation.

To add salt to Sabin's wounds, a very close personal relationship had formed between the top man at the NFIP, Basil O'Connor, and Salk, effectively leaving Sabin, emotionally at least, out in the cold.

Salk insists that throughout his whole association with polio research his aims were completely misunderstood. "I was not 'working on a vaccine for polio.' I was not 'working on a vaccine for influenza.' I was using the influenza and polio viruses to explore the possibilities of dissociating infectivity and antigenicity. . . . I could have done the same sort of thing with the tobacco mosaic virus or some animal virus."

However, like it or not, Salk could not "dissociate" himself from the great public concern with polio and his ultimate identification with all the developments surrounding the introduction of a vaccine. Such a vaccine promised to remove the menace that was threatening every American family at a seemingly increasing rate each year. At times the public uproar and the media attention gave rise to a circus atmosphere. Some of this would inevitably rub off on Salk.

At one point prior to the major field trial of Salk's vaccine, a perceptive virologist at the Rockefeller Institute, Frank Horsfall, commented to Rivers that Salk was in a no-win situation.

"If the vaccine fails it will be a black mark against him, but if it succeeds he'll be ruined. It's affixed to him and he to it."

Rivers recalled, "We could see that success, if it came, would make a public god out of him, distorting the meaning of his work, crediting him with achievements that belonged to Enders and Bodian and so many others and lousing him up with other scientists. We could see it [but] it was not our headache. Our job was to get a reasonably promising vaccine and see that it was tested properly."

The prediction was accurate, and Salk has had to live with the animosity of his colleagues ever since.

The Salk Institute in La Jolla is an aesthetic delight. The concrete main structure, set on high ground overlooking the Pacific, is modern in design. Its central court contains a reflecting pool and flowing fountain, and at lunchtime laboratory workers relax along the perimeters, brown bagging it in the sun and gentle breezes of Southern California. On each side of the court, the jagged facade presents several floors of windowed studies with a spectacular vista of blue sea and sky for the occupants.

It was Salk's own idea for "an experiment in the sociology of science," an attempt to foster creativity in an ideal environment, and he was intimately involved with the planning, design, and construction of the institute. It was founded in 1960, with the land donated by the city of San Diego. The March of Dimes (the fund-raising component of the NFIP) provided capital for construction to the tune of one million dollars annually over a ten-year period. To support the activities within, it also supplied a grant of a million dollars per year indefinitely, with the expectation that future grants obtained by members of the Salk Institute would replace these funds in later years. Temporary quarters were occuppied in 1963, and the permanent facility was ready for use in 1965. It has prospered.

A secretary leads me into a spacious, light oak-paneled room with west-facing windows at the far end. At one side of Dr. Salk's office is an oversized desk; opposite it is a sofa and coffee table where this rare interview will take place.

Dr. Salk enters. At seventy-three he still retains that aura of intensity, and the figure is still trim although a single curl of white encircles the nape of the neck. The initial response is polite but sober, guarded, suspicious. "Just what are you about? What exactly are you after?" Then the telephone rings, and he crosses the room to his desk to speak with one of his associates. The stiffness suddenly vanishes, a radiant smile lights up his face and a belly laugh, of which a moment before one had believed him incapable, emerges. The initial results of their experiment have been "marvelous." It looks like they're on the right track. He returns once more to the interview, and the pall descends. For all his success, when Salk talks about polio the tone is strangely resentful and heavy with regret. It is in startling contrast to the bright and uplifting surroundings.

Salk has never eclipsed the accomplishments of his earlier years with influenza and poliomyelitis, and, in all fairness, is it

justified to even broach the question? In science, medical or
otherwise, any investigator is fortunate to make even one important contribution to the body of our knowledge, and Salk
has more than realized this goal. There are rarities, those such
as Pasteur, Einstein, and Linus Pauling, who continued to per-
colate with new and exciting ideas throughout a long lifetime
of research. However, most scientists, even the best, often
make their most telling marks in their youth. Later on they
serve to foster the careers of others and provide a source of
experience and mature judgment upon which public policy
might be based.

At his institute, Salk's role has, to a great degree, been that
of enabling others to pursue their research interests, and a
number of Nobel Laureates—Francis Crick, Roger Guillemin,
and Renato Delbecco, for example—have found an environment conducive to their work. The late philosopher-mathe-
matician Jacob Bronowski, a fellow there in the early 1970s,
will be remembered for his moving book and television series
The Ascent of Man.

Salk has found some time for his own research interests,
studies in multiple sclerosis, and now has become involved in
the problem of AIDS. At this late stage of his career, he may
still have some significant contributions to make to a new and
increasingly menacing viral threat.

Sabin's life, devoted to the exploration of disease, has been
no stranger to the major incursions of illness upon it. In 1983
a paralyzing virus, of all things, still unidentified, totally im-
mobilized him for nearly six months. This strange illness was
punctuated by a cardiac arrest followed by a triple coronary
bypass operation. Added to this have come the onset of diabetes, prostate problems, and recurrent urinary tract infections which have taken their toll. Pressure on the spinal cord
from degenerative disk disease continues to threaten additional disability. Yet he remains acutely aware that the bless-
ings of his science have not yet been bestowed equally upon all
of God's children.

Although preventable by vaccination, there occur throughout the world each year nearly half a million cases of paralytic polio, two and a half million deaths from measles and its complications, and nearly another two million deaths from neonatal tetanus and pertussis (whooping cough). All this in tiny children, he observes, who have not yet had a chance to really live.

For these reasons, upon his recent return from a survey of immunization programs in Cuba and Nicaragua, Sabin, entering his ninth decade, still sees his work as largely unfinished.

Of Birds and Blood Cells

Bruce Glick Unravels the Secret of the Bursa of Fabricius

Nature study classes with Miss Hildebrand were always very special for the fourth graders at Pittsburgh's Whiteman Street School. She would often stop by at the Carnegie Museum to borrow a stuffed bird to demonstrate to her students. Tours through the neighboring streets to identify local species were often part of the program, and visits to the museum itself to view the feathered specimens on display were a highlight of such activities.

One youngster, Bruce Glick, was especially transfixed by this exposure to the world of birds. One day, shortly following one of these sessions after a severe storm had deposited a rare visitor, an American bittern, on the roof of his family garage, Bruce reached an important and irrevocable decision: he would devote the rest of his life to the study of birds.[1]

After growing into young manhood, completing high school, and serving in the army during World War II, Bruce enrolled in Rutgers University in 1947 as a science major to pursue his goal. Much to his dismay, however, he found that avian study in that particular academic environment consisted entirely of bird watching. In his own personal observations of bird life, he had already identified more than two hundred species. There was nothing new that this course work could offer him. What he really wanted to do was to work with birds, get inside them, examine them, discover what it was that made them function.

The only way to do this at Rutgers was to transfer to the Poultry Science Department. But the initial interview was not too promising. All of those ordinarily accepted by Professor Thompson, the head of the department, were farm boys. He informed Bruce, "It is one thing to be on the outside of a farm and looking in and quite another to be on the inside looking out." Thompson felt that a "city slicker" like Bruce might find himself out of place in such a program. The young man was insistent, however, and finally, after promising to spend the summer between his junior and senior years working on a farm, he was accepted as a transfer student into the Poultry Science Department. At last he would have the hands-on experience he craved.

While still an undergraduate at Rutgers, he began to study bird physiology under a pioneer in that field, Dr. Paul Sturkie. By the time he left Rutgers, however, Glick was primarily interested in population genetics, which he pursued for a year at Amherst, gaining his master's degree in the process. This distraction was only temporary; the early 1950s found him again involved in bird study, this time as a graduate student at Ohio State's agricultural college. But the beginnings there could hardly be called auspicious. Under Professor R. George Jaap, he was assigned a research project for which he could develop no enthusiasm whatsoever, and his progress report to Jaap clearly reflected this. While grappling with this unpromising project one evening, Glick took a break from his studies and wandered into the basement laboratory of the facility. There he found his professor at the dissection table bent over the body of a goose. In one hand he held an odd saclike structure that his student had never seen before. His curiosity piqued, Glick inquired, "What is that?"

"It is called the bursa of Fabricius."

"What is its function?"

"That's a good question. Why don't you find the answer?"

The course of Glick's life and, indeed, that of the science of immunology would be altered by this brief exchange.

Hieronymus Fabricius (Giralamo Fabrici, 1533–1619) was one of a line of brilliant anatomists, physicians, and surgeons at Padua, which flourished among other northern Italian medical schools during the sixteenth century.[2] Vesalius, perhaps the most preeminent anatomist of all time, taught there. He was succeeded by his student, Gabriele Fallopio (after whom the ovaries' fallopian tubes were named), who in turn taught Fabricius. The latter numbered among his many accomplishments the instruction of William Harvey, who would first accurately describe the circulation of the blood following his return to England. Harvey even lived for a period as part of Fabricius's household in Padua and used some of his mentor's plates in the publication of his own work.

Among the many studies Fabricius performed was one in which he described in chickens the saccular gland that bears his name. For more than four hundred years anatomists and embryologists had observed this gland in many species of birds, but had never come up with a good explanation of exactly what it did and why. In the chicken, the urogenital and digestive tracts merge toward their termination to form a common chamber, the cloaca. It is from this that the saclike bursa protrudes before gradually regressing and disappearing in adult life. Fabricius had postulated that it served as a storage place for semen, but this could never be substantiated.

It was Glick's failure to progress satisfactorily with his assigned research that stimulated him, about a month after his late-hours encounter with his professor, to consider looking into the matter of the bursa of Fabricius. A visit to the library revealed only a few studies—most in Italian or French—and none very enlightening. It seemed a potentially fruitful area to investigate.

Glick first began to study the natural history of the gland in the chicken and found that it grew most rapidly during the first three weeks of life, then reaching a plateau at about two months before regressing and disappearing completely by the end of the first year. He then studied the effects of various hormones on bursal growth. Finally, he utilized the classical approach to the study of glandular function—remove the gland and then observe the effects on the animal.

Previous workers had removed the gland at about the fourth week after hatching or later. Glick's observations about the early rapid growth of the gland led him to perform these bursectomies at a much earlier stage, prior to the twelfth day of life. Despite this early intervention, subsequent analysis of various aspects of development and function (growth rates, feathering, and so on) demonstrated no obvious effects of the gland's extirpation. Could it be that in the modern-day chick it no longer had any function at all?

Glick's pondering over his experiments had to await the chance intercession of another graduate student, Timothy Chang, before he would stumble over the real significance of his work. Chang, who was involved mainly in poultry pathology, was assigned to demonstrate an antigen-antibody reaction to a class of undergraduate students. The laboratory exercise was a simple and practical field test to demonstrate resistance to a particular infection. It involved first the injection into a group of chickens of an inactivated bacterium, *Salmonella pullorum*. A week would be allowed for the development of antibodies in the chickens. They would then be returned to the laboratory. In preparation for this, glass warming plates would be prepared with a stained antigen that had been extracted from laboratory cultures of the bacteria. When a drop of blood from an immunized chicken was placed on a warming plate, illuminated from below by a light, the antibodies produced as a result of the previous inoculation would combine with the antigen, forming agglutinated colored clumps, visible to the naked eye.

Chang's immediate problem was that he had no animals available with which he could make this demonstration. He turned to his friend Glick, whom he knew kept dozens of chickens on tap for his own experiments, and asked if he could borrow a few for this purpose. Glick agreed to make them available.

At the initial laboratory session, Chang performed the inoculations before the gathered students and informed them that, a week later, he would return with the chickens and demonstrate the antigen-antibody reaction described. When the time arrived, Chang withdrew some blood from the first chicken and placed a drop on the warming plate which contained the stained salmonella antigen. Nothing. He tried a second. Nothing. Then a third, with the same result. One can imagine the mischievous delight of the students as the confident demeanor of their instructor dissolved into confusion. In all, 80 percent of the chickens failed to demonstrate the antigen-antibody reaction, just the opposite of what had been the predicted result.

A distraught Chang confronted Glick with the results of this fiasco. They checked the tags of all the chicks used in the experiment. The nonresponders had all been previously bursectomized. Only the sham-operated animals, those surgically opened and closed without the bursa removal and used by Glick as controls for his own experiments, had developed antibodies as predicted. It appeared clear that the removal of a bursa had resulted in failure of the chicks to develop circulating antibodies to infection.

Glick and Chang then embarked on a systematic study of the effect of bursectomy. In more than a hundred birds of differing breeds and in both sexes, the results were the same. No bursa, no antibodies. Curiously, the excitement of the two graduate students was not fully shared by their respective professors. Nonetheless, Jaap agreed to help Glick write up the results for his first scientific report, and the paper was submitted to the prestigious journal *Science*.

By this time, Glick was reaching the end of his tenure at Ohio State and was off to an interview for a junior faculty position at Mississippi State University. (He was offered the job, accepted it, and has spent most of his professional life there.) In his absence from Ohio State, a rejection letter arrived from *Science*. It was suggested therein that "further elucidation of the mechanism . . . should be attempted before publication." Over the telephone, Jaap suggested to Glick that he could, with a minor alteration in format, prepare the report for the journal *Poultry Science*, and the latter agreed.[3]

Recently, regarding the rejection of *Science* and its suggestion for elucidation of mechanism, Glick has noted that ultimately this would require several years and "the resources of, at least, nine laboratories in the United States and Canada, and major laboratories in Australia, Austria, England, Finland, France, Germany, Italy, Japan, Sweden and Yugoslavia." The article in *Poultry Science* has since been selected as a citation classic in the literature of science.

At the time, the report in the obscure poultry journal might have gone completely unnoticed by the medical community. As one physician later put it, "Who the hell reads *Poultry Science?*" Fortunately, Harold Wolfe did. Wolfe was a professor of zoology at the University of Wisconsin whose research involved the immunology of chickens. When he saw the article by Glick, Chang, and Jaap, he recognized its potential importance to a physician friend of his, Bob Good, who was vitally interested in just such phenomena.

Robert A. Good, an M.D.-Ph.D. at the University of Minnesota, had committed himself to the developing field of immunology ever since his graduation from medical school in the early post-World War II years.[4] After completing his formal pediatric training in 1949 at the University of Minnesota, he spent a year at the Rockefeller Institute in New York. Part of his work took him to the bedsides of certain patients in the adjacent Sloan-Kettering Cancer Institute. There he was impressed by some striking differences in susceptibility to infections in two types of cancer patients. Those with Hodgkin's lymphomas, he found, often fell victims to tuberculosis, fungal infections, and certain viral infections. They rarely came down with infections due to bacteria such as the pneumococcus, streptococus, and pseudomonas. Conversely, patients with multiple myeloma, a disease in which the proliferation of abnormal plasma cells is the hallmark, showed exactly the opposite pattern of proclivity to infection. Good recalls, "So here we had two groups of patients with hematopoietic malignancies with totally different susceptibilities to infections. It was this that first got me to thinking about the possibility of there being two different types of cell lines separable for immunity and two major bulwarks against infections. I began, through a haze, to see these experiments of nature dissecting the microbial universe."[5]

There had been some hints about the thymus gland having some role in immunity, and Good and his associates had been performing thymectomies in experimental animals to determine the effect of this gland on resistance to infection. There had thus far been little in the way of positive results. His reading of Glick's paper, describing early bursectomies, suggested to him that he and his coworkers had been performing their thymectomies too late in the life cycle of their mice and rats, and they began to perform the thymectomies in the newborn period, with demonstrable effects on the development of certain kinds of immunity later in life.

Those blood elements we ordinarily call "white cells" because of their appearance as a fluffy layer a millimeter or so thick between the red cells and plasma in a tube of centrifuged blood consist predominantly of three types. The first, comprising about 50 to 70 percent of the total, are called polymorphonuclear cells ("polys") because of the odd-shaped nucleus—the center, resembling a multilobed pawnbroker's insignia. These are our first line of defense against microbial intruders, gobbling up any they recognize within the blood stream.

The second type is the monocyte, larger than the "poly" but not as numerous (5 to 10 percent of the total). It is also present in the tissues, where it is called a macrophage ("big eater"). Monocytes can also kill unwelcome visitors, frequently communicating with other parts of the immunologic system in the process.

The third type, the lymphocytes, comprise 25 to 30 percent of the circulating white cells, and it is they that are the main actors in the story of the bursa. Lymphoid cells, we now know, originate in the bone marrow. From there, they mainly take one of two developmental routes: one will convert them into T lymphocytes; the other will produce B lymphocytes.

The T lymphocytes are those processed through the thymus gland, located in the center of the chest right behind the breast bone. When mature, these cells are directly involved in such immune reactions as those concerning resistance to certain infections (for example, tuberculosis). They are also the cells responsible for graft rejection, contact allergies, and apparently the killing of some cancer cells.

The B lymphocytes (after the bursa of Fabricius), although completely indistinguishable on a stained blood smear slide from their cousins in the T line, have a different spectrum of activity. They are responsible for the production of circulating antibodies (immunogloblulins in nature) either directly, in small amounts, or by developing into plasma cells, superproducers of antibody. The reason that Good's patients at Sloan-Kettering were susceptible to different types of infection had to do with the deficiency or inadequate function of the particular type of lymphocyte involved. Incidentally, there is no recognizable bursa such as that of Fabricius in humans. It is believed that human B cell transformation occurs before birth in the fetal liver.

To return to our story, the first practical applications of all this knowledge about lymphocyte differentiation did not occur directly in the field of infectious disease, but rather within the somewhat rarified group of inherited immunodeficiency diseases that Good and other pediatric specialists began to recognize among their patients.

Some of these children lacked functional B cells; others could not produce T cells. The most devastating of these disorders was severe combined immunodeficiency disease, a sexlinked genetically transmitted disorder in which neither T nor B cells were produced in the affected males, resulting in their early deaths from overwhelming infection.

In 1967, one such boy was brought to Good, who attempted to correct the deficiency with the transplantation of fetal liver cells. A fatal graft-*versus*-host reaction developed. That is, the transplanted cells recognized the boy's normal tissues as foreign and attacked them. Despite this failure, Good and his colleagues were convinced of the basic validity of their approach. A child born without a functioning thymus gland had already received a thymus transplant elsewhere and survived in good health.

Their second chance came a year later when David Camp, a little boy from Meriden, Connecticut, was brought to Minnesota. He had severe combined immunodeficiency disease, and the future was bleak. Twelve male members of his family had already died from the disease, and, without treatment, David would surely be the thirteenth. As his physicians pondered the correct approach to take, they were haunted by the memory of the previous graft-*versus*-host reaction in their first patient. Would a bone marrow transplant be more likely to succeed than that of fetal liver obtained from a stillborn premature birth?

One night the idea came to Good that what they must do was use a bone marrow transplant from a sibling of David's, one who would be perfectly matched immunologically. Statistically, there was one chance in four that any sibling would fit the bill, and David had four sisters as potential donors. With the relatively crude tissue-matching techniques of the day, they determined that none of these was actually a perfect match, although one girl, Doreen, was the closest. The bone marrow transplant took, but again a graft-*versus*-host reaction took place, and Doreen's transplanted cells began to destroy all of David's other blood cells. He rapidly developed an aplastic anemia. The next step was untried previously but proved to be an inspired one. The Minnesota team, rather than removing Doreen's transplant, performed a second one. The blood cells from this second transplant took hold and began rapidly to populate the barren stretches of bone marrow that awaited them. They have remained there, functioning normally ever since.

Such were the initial payoffs of the burgeoning knowledge to which discoveries such as Glick's contributed. Today it is recognized that the original simple division into "T cells" and "B cells" is inadequate to describe the whole system. There have been subdivisions into T helper cells (victims of the AIDS virus), T suppressor cells, "killer" cells, natural and otherwise. Immunological aspects of a variety of other previously poorly understood diseases have been recognized. Useful classifications of various lymphomas have been derived through immunological techniques leading to more rational approaches to evaluation and treatment. Finally, through the use of monoclonal antibodies, another outgrowth of immunological research, new ways are being found to detect many cancers early and perhaps eradicating them as well.

The recognition of T and B lymphocyte subgroups has, perhaps, achieved even greater importance with the emergence of AIDS as an increasing worldwide threat. Although macrophages have recently been implicated as targets of the retrovirus causing AIDs, it was the T lymphocyte that was first recognized as a primary victim of HIV (human immunodeficiency virus). Thanks to the work of Glick and Good, this discovery provided scientists with initial routes for investigation of the pathogenesis of the disease and, it is hoped, its ultimate control.

Throughout all these developments, Glick, now at Clemson University, has continued his immunological and physiological investigations, maintaining an intense interest in the bursa of Fabricius. His eyes lighting up, he notes that in the kiwi bird of New Zealand the bursa survives intact throughout its life, and he would love to study the biological implications of that persistence.

As for his initial work on the bursa, Glick recalls that his discovery owed a great deal to the salmonella bacterium that Chang had selected for his laboratory exercise. It turns out that, among the infinite number of substances to which a chick might develop immunity, antibodies to *S. pullorum* develop rather late in relation to hatching date. Thus the bursectomies performed during the first two weeks of life were able to prevent the normal immunological resistance that would have otherwise taken place. Had another "bug" been chosen, one to which antibodies developed much earlier, perhaps even prior to hatching, Chang's demonstration would have gone off without a hitch. It would have been a complete "success"—and to this day the secret of the bursa might remain unrevealed.

A Plague in Philadelphia

The Story of Legionnaires' Disease

On November 18, 1976, Philadelphia's Bellevue-Stratford Hotel was forced to close its doors.[1] The events there over the preceding four months had frightened the public to such an extent that no one dared any longer to enter the once popular stopping place for tourists, business people, and others passing through the City of Brotherly Love.

The growing panic leading to this event would never have occurred if it had been a traveling salesman, an isolated government worker, or a foreign tourist who had been taken ill following a stay at the Philadelphia landmark. But in the summer of 1976, more than four thousand Pennsylvanians attended the Fifty-eighth Annual Convention of its American Legion Department there between July 21 and 24. In the succeeding days, as one after another of this group became deathly ill, it became apparent that something had gone terribly wrong within and about the environs of the hotel.

Those afflicted, ultimately 221 individuals, were typically stricken with high unremitting fevers, chills, and general prostration. Clinical and X-ray findings revealed the lungs to be the major target organ. Only this was clear at first. The subsequent events involving the investigation and discovery of this new malady provide a paradigm for all those concerned with the maintenance of the public's health and for the rest of us dependent on them for our protection.

Although many individuals both at the Centers for Disease Control (CDC) in Atlanta as well as at the Pennsylvania State Department of Health contributed to the defining of what we have come to call Legionnaires' disease, two individuals have become most identified with it: Dr. David W. Fraser, an epidemiologist from CDC who headed the field team assigned to the outbreak; and Dr. Joseph E. McDade, the microbiologist at CDC who finally identified the causative organism. Their respective activities in the field and at home base in Atlanta easily suggest the terminology once applied to West Point's football heroes of the mid-1940s, Glenn Davis and Felix "Doc" Blanchard: "Mr. Outside" and "Mr. Inside."

"Mr. Outside," Dr. Fraser, was one of the few graduates of the Harvard Medical School class of 1969 who was interested in epidemiology. The study and control of disease outbreaks among populations rather than individual illness is not the career goal of many graduating physicians. But Fraser found this fascinating and went for training to the CDC in Atlanta for a two-year stint as an Epidemic Intelligence Service officer to get the best experience available. This program of the CDC, then about thirty-five years in existence, had been set up originally to train physicians who might be involved in fighting biological warfare. As it turned out, developments in Philadelphia might well have been classified under "biological warfare."

In 1976, the CDC was broadly divided into two sections: the Bureau of Laboratories and the Bureau of Epidemiology. Fraser, after having completed his training at CDC, with additional experience in internal medicine and infectious disease work at the University of Pennsylvania Medical School, had returned to Atlanta and was assigned to the Special Pathogen Branch. The CDC, then and now, is set up to assist state health departments in dealing with various public health problems as they arise, and EIS officers such as Fraser were equally divided in their assignments to Atlanta or one of the state health departments. Recognition of an emergent problem can arise at either the state or federal level, and the two arms of public health often operate in tandem.

In this instance, Fraser recalls, Atlanta received its first notice of the new disease early on Monday morning, August 2. A call was received from a Veterans Administration clinic physician, who reported four deaths and some additional cases of nonfatal pneumonia among veterans who had attended the recent Legionnaires' convention in Philadelphia. He was immediately referred to the Influenza Surveillance Group. This was, after all, 1976, the year in which Asian flu had made its appearance, and a dreaded repeat of the 1918 pandemic was considered a distinct possibility. Those familiar with that earlier episode had good reason to fear a new outbreak. The mortality figures back then had approached those of the Black Death in fourteenth-century London. At this point in the investigation, influenza was high on their list of possibilities, and already those stricken with the disease had demonstrated an alarming mortality. Later that same Monday, when a CDC official called back the VA physician for clarification, he was informed of an additional eleven deaths that had surfaced since that morning. Something "special" was surely going on in Pennsylvania.

The Pennsylvania state health department was by this time already on the job and welcomed the CDC's assistance. Although the outbreak could be traced to Philadelphia, the conventioners had, by this time, returned to their homes all over the state. With teams operating out of Harrisburg and Pittsburgh as well as Philadelphia, more than twenty EIS officers from the CDC, with David Fraser assigned to head them, joined scores of state health workers in the massive task of examining and interviewing each case and collecting specimens of blood, sputum, and urine from the living as well as tissue samples from the affected organs of the dead. All of these specimens were divided in half by the state and shared with the laboratory service of the CDC in Atlanta.

As it turned out, most of the patients involved became ill between July 22 and August 3; by the end of the first week of August the outbreak was essentially over. But this could not be known during the first few days of the emergency, and, given the mysteriousness of the disease, panic quickly began to set in.

Fraser, at first based in Harrisburg, describes the mayhem already surrounding him on the second day of the investigation, Tuesday, August 3. He would be sitting at a desk in the state health department trying to keep up with an unending stream of telephone inquiries with a reporter perched at either end of his desk, plying him with additional questions each time a phone call had been completed. "It was" he recalls, "an environment in which it was hard to do science—or anything else!"

The following day, the state secretary of health sequestered Fraser in another building to shield him and his assistants from the constant barrage of questions. Thereafter, press conferences were held twice daily, and they were able to get on with the work at hand.

At the end of the first week of August, when the number of new cases clearly began to drop off sharply, Fraser moved his team to Philadelphia to try to sort things out.

What did they know? By the end of the outbreak, a total of 221 people had become ill; seventy-two of them were not even Legionnaires. However, they were all either in the hotel or out on the sidewalk adjoining it ("Broad Street pneumonia") preceding the episode. The disease varied from a mild grippelike illness to a severe pneumonia, with thirty-four ultimately dying from either the lung disease or its complications. Those coming down with the disease were more likely to be older than those who did not, tended to be smokers and also males, with a three-to-one sex ratio.

What had caused the disease, and what was the mode of transmission? It would be months before the first question could be answered because all the initial specimen examinations were failing to identify a recognizable agent. As for the second question, the extensive fieldwork that had been performed was at least somewhat helpful in ruling in or out various possibilities. The disease did not seem to have been spread from person to person; food contamination was unlikely; the possibility of an insect vector was also discarded. It remained possible that the disease could have been either airborne or related to some form of water contamination, but no hard evidence was at hand. Fraser and his assistants had spent

hours scurrying about the air ducts of the hotel without un-
covering a clue.

On August 20, still with no clear idea of what it was that had
caused the outbreak, Fraser and his team returned to Atlanta
to prepare the first draft of their field report, which was to be
completed in November.

There is an old motto among epidemiologists: always arrive
after the epidemic has peaked; otherwise you'll be blamed for
failing to stop it. The CDC, including Fraser and his coworkers, were soon to become painfully aware of the truth of
this, having been on the scene so early and having failed to
come up with the right answers.

Although professionals in the field could find no fault with
their procedures, this provided little comfort as public criticism mounted. Joseph A. Califano, secretary for health, education, and welfare, reported to the press that, as a result of
his conversations with health professionals all over the country, his impression was that the CDC had slipped; it was not
the first-rate outfit it used to be. Dr. David J. Sencer, director
of the CDC, who had received an award for excellence from
the Public Health Association only a year earlier, was now suspected of not having a firm grip on things.

Congress got into the act. In November 1976, the Con-
sumer Protection Subcommittee of the House Judiciary Committee convened hearings on the matter. Its chairman,
Representative John M. Murphy (whose image of rectitude,
incidentally, would later be shattered by his bribery conviction
in the Abscam investigation), criticized the CDC for their "mis-
direction of resources . . . their tunnel vision toward swine flu
. . . lack of organization." The final subcommittee report accused the CDC of "bungling and ineptitude" and, as a result
of their own independent investigation, concluded that an unknown toxic substance was the cause of the disease that had
attacked the Philadelphia conventioneers.

The best the CDC could do at the time was to say what the
disease was *not*. It had *not* been influenza virus. It had *not* been
bubonic plague or typhoid fever; or lymphocytic choriomen-
ingitis or parrot fever; or whooping cough or tularemia. Their

sense of frustration at this point was best expressed by Dr. Robert Sharrar, then chief of the CDC's Communicable Disease Control Section attached to the Philadelphia Department of Health. "We may never know what caused Legionnaires' disease. We did everything possible but we're not God. We may never know."

In the wake of these doubts and inability to identify a microbial pathogen as the cause of the disease, a host of hypotheses arose and experts were called in to wrestle with them.

Could fluorocarbons used as refrigerants in the hotel cooling system have been the culprits? Had a herbicide, paraquat, somehow managed to get into the drinking water? The symptoms of some victims resembled those of nickel carbonyl poisoning, and nickel traces had been found in the lung specimens of some who had succumbed to the disease. Was this the answer? Could the affected Legionnaires have imbibed moonshine whiskey that had been contaminated with ethylene glycol? Was there a new virus on the scene?

The Franklin Institute was called in to reinvestigate the air conditioning system and cooling ducts but to no avail. The Academy of Natural Sciences looked into the water supply. Drexel University performed mass spectrometry and other sophisticated laboratory tests on water specimens obtained. At the Bellevue Stratford nineteen separate violations of the city plumbing code were detected, but these still could not explain the epidemic. Physicists at Harvard and the Massachusetts Institute of Technology examined hair specimens of the survivors in the search for clues to an intermittent exposure to some toxic substance in the air. The University of Connecticut examined the nickel poisoning hypothesis and concluded that it was likely a contaminant from the knives used to prepare lung tissue specimens for the pathologists after similar nickel traces had been found in the lungs of autopsied patients who had not been victims of the disease.

Meanwhile, three experts from the National Institute of Occupational Safety and Health were consulted about the possibility of industrial poisons and the adequacy of industrial hygiene at the site. Dr. Alexander D. Langmuir, the respected

former head of epidemiology at the CDC, was called out of
retirement for his opinion. His only contribution was that this
was "the greatest epidemiological puzzle of the century."

Finally, a twelve-man committee of infectious disease specialists, bolstered by a panel of eight internationally acclaimed
pathologists, were asked for their evaluation. Of one thing
only could they all be certain, they concluded: they did not
know what had caused the epidemic, but, whatever it was, it
was *not* a bacterium. The validity of that particular judgment
would finally be tested back at the CDC. For this aspect of the
story, we must turn to the growing involvement of Mr. Inside, Dr. Joseph E. McDade, a microbiologist there, back in
Atlanta.

The Centers for Disease Control looms large in the consciousness of American medicine. In addition to its forays into
the field to investigate ongoing and potential health problems,
the agency keeps a running scorecard on the nation's health.
Through its weekly *Morbidity and Mortality Report,* published in
the widely disseminated *Journal of the American Medical Association,* and other health bulletins emanating from Atlanta, this
governmental agency keeps the medical community abreast of
current advances as well as possible danger points within the
health care scene both at home and abroad.

Despite its preeminence, the CDC presents itself to the visitor as a rather unprepossessing collection of low-lying build-
ings on the outskirts of Atlanta, adjoining the campus of
Emory University. As one enters its maze of corridors, ramps
and stairways, it becomes immediately apparent that func-
tionalism rather than architectural excellence was uppermost
in the minds of the builders. Along one corridor, flanked on
the left by a bank of windows overlooking a drab courtyard, a
door opens on the right to a secretarial office-anteroom. This,
in turn, leads to another windowless cubicle, the office of Joseph E. McDade. A desk is pushed flush against the far wall
upon which two enlarged photographs are hung. Immediately
above the desk is a large colored photographic poster of an
old section of Cumberland, Maryland. Featured in the lower
right-hand corner is a grocery store with a large sign reading

"McDade's." Higher on the wall to the left is an eight-by-ten-inch enlarged photomicrograph of the rod-shaped bacterium we have come to know as *Legionella pneumophila.*

Joe McDade, now in his midforties, is a balding, blondish, soft-spoken man with a brush moustache. He recalls that it was an unusual set of coincidences that fell into place as he was confronted with the problem of Legionnaires' disease ten years earlier when he had barely arrived at CDC to assume his job as the new rickettsiologist "on the block."

But first, to understand the dilemma that faced these medical investigators and appreciate their initial frustration, it is important to know something about the microbial world accounting for the infectious diseases with which they must deal on a daily basis.

In terms of size, at the larger end of the spectrum and visible under the light microscope, are the bacteria that cause many of the lung, skin, and urinary tract infections to which humans are susceptible. Although these microorganisms were among the other "animalcules" seen as early as 1677 by Antony van Leeuwenhoek, inventor of the microscope, their clear connection with disease was not made until two hundred years later. At that time, Robert Koch, then a young district medical officer in Silesia (now part of Poland), identified the anthrax bacillus in the blood of sheep that had become infected. Koch later identified a number of other pathogens, including the one causing tuberculosis. On the basis of his experience, he introduced his famous postulates for identifying a disease-causing microorganism.

- First, the organism should regularly be found in the lesions of the disease.
- Second, it must be isolated in pure culture.
- Third, inoculation of the cultured organisms should cause a similar disease in an experimental animal.
- Fourth, the organism must be recovered from the lesions produced in the laboratory animal.

These postulates were regularly met for a variety of bacterial diseases studies subsequently, and for many diseases under current study they may still prove quite valid, especially those caused by bacteria. To help researchers and physicians detect these organisms in body fluids and pathological tissue specimens, certain dyes were developed which are preferentially taken up by the microbes, making them stand out in various colors on the slides prepared for inspection.

At the smallest end of the microbial spectrum lie the viruses (from the Latin for "poison"). Although it was long suspected that microorganisms too small to be visualized under the light microscope might be the cause of a number of diseases—as indeed they are, with polio, smallpox, infectious hepatitis, and the common cold being only a few examples—it was not until the 1930s, when the electron microscope was invented, that these tiny particles could actually be visualized. Viruses differ from bacteria in another way: they cannot be cultured on plates containing artificial media. They will survive and multiply only within living cells.

The rickettsiae occupy a place midway between the other two categories of microbes. In size they resemble small bacteria, although they require different staining techniques to make them readily visible on the microscopic slide. But, like the viruses, they will grow only within living susceptible tissue. Rickettsiae account for a much smaller number of human diseases than bacteria and viruses and were not recognized until 1906 when a Chicago pathologist identified one type as the cause of Rocky Mountain spotted fever. In 1910, he and an associated traveled to Mexico to investigate an outbreak of disease that also turned out to be rickettsial in nature, epidemic typhus. On this occasion, however, he became infected with the disease himself and died later that year. The contributions of Howard T. Ricketts are memorialized in the name given to the new types of organisms he was the first to describe.

By the early 1970s, the study of rickettsial disease was not looked upon as the leading-edge research for aspiring microbiologists. Most of the work in the field had been accomplished in the preceding decades, and many of those who had toiled in those particular vineyards of research were already retired or certainly on the verge.

Joe McDade was not born a rickettsiologist; he had made no

effort to achieve this status; it was, more or less, thrust upon him. Coming of college age in the recession years of the mid-1950s, McDade was initially inclined toward arts and letters, but his parents were unable to finance his college education. His childless uncle, however, owner of a prosperous grocery store, offered to assist him as long as he applied himself to a more practical field. Starting off as a premedical student at Western Maryland College, Joe later gravitated toward more basic biological problems, eventually earning his masters degree and Ph.D. in microbiology at the University of Delaware.

To fulfill his ROTC obligations during the 1960s, McDade entered the army and was assigned to the biological laboratories at Fort Detrick, where a vacancy for a rickettsiologist existed. With no previous experience in the field, he was ordered to fill it. This first brush with rickettsiae led, among other scientific efforts, to fieldwork in Egypt and Ethiopia to study outbreaks of typhus. Returning from Africa in 1975, he learned that the CDC wished to set up a new rickettsial section in Atlanta. All the older men in the field were gone. He was invited to accept the position and did.

At the beginning of the investigation of the Philadelphia outbreak, McDade had been at the CDC for only eight months. Like the rest of the nation, he was, or course, aware of the problem, but he was involved only peripherally inasmuch as the disease was so clearly unrickettsial in nature. The incubation period was just a day or two before the clinical manifestations became apparent. In rickettsial infections, incubation took a week or so. The early onset of symptoms following apparent exposure favored a bacterial cause, whereas some of the clinical manifestations suggested a virus. Nobody's money was on the rickettsiae, which kept McDade out of the picture.

However, as time passed, with the failure to incriminate any of the more likely pathogens, more thought was given to the possibility of a rickettsial etiology. Uppermost in the minds of the CDC investigators was the possibility of Q Fever (after "query," denoting originally that the cause was unknown). Q

Fever occasionally included pneumonia among its manifestations, and although death was rare in Q Fever and proving rather common in Legionnaires' disease, McDade was asked to rule it out.

To appreciate fully the difficulties encountered by McDade and understand the course of his investigations that finally led to the solution, the reader might be aided at the outset by three aspects of this bacterial disease that confounded the initial efforts to identity it:

- Pathologically, the pneumonia caused by the *Legionella* organism resembles that caused by a virus rather than the typical bacterial pneumonia.
- The stains used on tissues, sputum slides, etc., which are almost invariably taken up by other bacteria are not taken up by the *Legionella* organism. Thus, this bacterium does not stain like other bacteria.
- The culture media used to grow a wide spectrum of other bacteria failed to meet the metabolic requirements of the fastidious *Legionella*. Attempts with as many as fifteen or twenty different types of media were uniformly unsuccessful.

In brief, then, this bacterium did not stain like a bacterium; it did not grow like other bacteria; and the disease it caused resembled that caused by viruses much more than bacterial infections.

The steps taken by McDade in his search for a rickettsial organism differed somewhat from the classical approach of Koch, given the nature of the microbe he was hunting. There are two ways to identify a rickettsial species, one direct and one indirect.

The direct approach involves using suspensions of infected material obtained from victims of the disease, and inoculating them into a laboratory animal such as a guinea pig or another living host convenient for laboratory work, a fertilized ("embryonated") chicken egg incubated in a warm nurturing environment. Within the susceptible host, the rickettsiae will then grow and later be isolated from the tissues of the victim for identification.

One indirect way of proving a rickettsial species as a cause of a disease is to utilize an antigen-antibody approach. Individuals who survive exposure to a certain pathogen form increasing numbers of antibodies to it as the disease runs its course. These are few in number early in the disease and plentiful following recovery (acute and convalescent phases). A rising number of antibodies to a particular pathogen, demonstrated by combining the patient's blood serum with the antigen and demonstrating the increasing evidence of antigen/antibody combinations, serves to prove that pathogen to have been the cause of the disease.

McDade started in a routine manner, using guinea pigs. These endearing little rodents serve the laboratory as wonderful biological filters in the isolation of rickettsiae. Pathological specimens are invariably contaminated with environmental bacteria by the time they are delivered to the laboratory to begin a search for rickettsiae. Fortunately, guinea pigs are remarkably resistant to most of these bacteria and, within a day or two, clear them from their bodies where the sought-for rickettsiae are now permitted to grow in relatively pure culture.

In this case, however, instead of the mild fever "blip" a day or two after inoculation, indicating the guinea pigs' elimination of the bacterial "contaminants," McDade's guinea pigs went on to develop an overwhelming febrile illness leading to their death within three or four days. Very unrickettsial, indeed.

McDade thought that they might have succumbed to a bacterial contaminant and, to rid himself of this complicating problem, tried passing the possibly infective material from the first guinea pig group through a second. This was not successful; no fever or any other signs of illness were observed during the second passage. He then decided to subculture suspensions of infected guinea pig spleen into embryonated eggs. To these he added a small amount of antibiotic, just enough, he hoped, to suppress the bacteria but not the rickettsiae. The embryonated eggs grew nothing.

The only clue to the ultimate solution at this time lay in the slides of the infected guinea pig tissue. Ordinary stains did

show collections of cocci (rounded forms of bacteria), and
some of these even grew on culture plates. But these could be
dismissed from consideration because they were identified as
nonpathogenic bacteria that are frequently seen in these animals. On a special stain for rickettsiae, the Gimenez technique,
he noticed a rare bacillus (rod-shaped form), but McDade was
inclined to doubt its significance. If bacteria were causing such
a devastating pneumonia, why were they not more plentiful?
And why would they not have grown out on one or more of
the numerous types of culture media? For all he knew, the few
bacilli he had seen may have dropped from someone's fingers
in the preparation of the slide.

At this point, McDade was sure he had done his job in ruling out a rickettsial cause for Legionnaires' disease. Furthermore, the most promising theory then being considered was
that the disease was not an infection after all, but related to
the toxic effects of nickel. In mid-September he dropped his
participation in the project and returned to other work awaiting his attention.

As the weeks passed and the nickel carbonyl theory petered
out, McDade's thoughts returned to his slides. The cocci he
had found had not troubled him, but those rare rod-shaped
forms kept nagging at him. The Monday between Christmas
and New Years is a quiet time to work, free of distractions and
interruptions. McDade returned to his laboratory, took out
the slide box, and extracted a guinea pig spleen slide for review. As chance would have it this time, instead of a rare rod-
shaped organism here and there, he found a cluster of them
being engulfed by a white blood cell. This indicated an active
infection going on rather than just a microbe in the vicinity
that had happened to drop on the plate.

Now he performed the critical laboratory maneuver. He
placed some of a suspension of infected guinea pig spleen into
some embryonated eggs, but this time omitted the addition of
antibiotic. Several days later the embryos were dead, and
when the yolk sac membranes were harvested and smears
treated with the Gimenez stain, an abundance of rod-shaped
organisms were immediately apparent under the microscope.

The final connection to the human Legionnaires' disease was made by testing blood sera saved at various stages of the disease against the organism isolated by McDade. This was done by a fluorescent antibody technique. Briefly, suspensions of infected yolk sac membranes containing the organism were placed on microscopic slides. Sera from patients containing antibodies to the organism were then added, the antibodies of the patients combining with the antigen proteins on the surface of the rods. To make this antigen-antibody complex visible under the microscope, a second antigen-antibody reaction was used. Antibodies from rabbits that had been made sensitized to human antibody (used in the rabbits as an antigen) were labeled with a fluorescent dye and added as a third component to the slides. The rabbit antibody attached to the human antibody/*Legionella* complex, forming clusters of glowing fluorescence when viewed under the microscope with ultraviolet light. The relative concentration of these antibodies could be verified by testing the sera at increasing dilutions. The amount of antibodies was found to increase between the early and late stages of the disease.

At this point, it was still not clear whether the disease-causing organism was a large rickettsial species or a small bacterium. This question was finally resolved in another CDC laboratory to which McDade sent samples of viable infected tissue. There specialists in the preparation of bacteriological culture media, much like master chefs, kept experimenting with the addition of various nutrients until they concocted a combination that finally satisfied the organism's curious appetite, one high in iron and the amino acid cysteine.

It could now be said with conviction that the cause of the disease was a bacterium and, in deference to those who were so prominently afflicted with it and the organ to which it showed such a pronounced predilection, the name *Legionella pneumophila* was proposed as the most appropriate.

When pressed as to the motivating force behind his persistence, McDade puts it this way, "The fact that the rods wouldn't grow bothered me. You have to account for everything you see."

He talks about a "matrix," a sort of epidemiological box score where all the possibilities are lined up on one axis and the things you have to do to rule them in or out on the other.

"Until you complete your matrix, your job is not done. It's different in pure research. There you follow the most promising leads, those that will probably give the results you seek, and sort of let the others go by. But when you're working for the public, you have an obligation to complete everything even if it's likely some of them will turn out to be 'red herrings'."

McDade was compelled to complete the matrix.[2]

There were additional payoffs from this discovery.[3] The CDC keeps records of past investigations that had failed to disclose the cause of a disease outbreak. The evidence pertaining to these failures are the stored frozen serum specimens from patients who had come down with the unknown disease. One such unresolved episode had occurred in Pontiac, Michigan eight years earlier, in 1968. After the discovery of *Legionella,* some senior people at CDC recognized similarities between what was called "Pontiac fever" and Legionnaires' disease. When the sera from the Pontiac patients was tested against *Legionella* by the fluorescent antibody technique, 85 percent proved positive.

In 1977, a new *Legionella* outbreak was documented in Burlington, Vermont, and investigators were now prepared to quickly recognize and deal with it. In 1978, Bloomington, Indiana, was the locus, and epidemics have been documented in places as distantly separated as Memphis, Tennessee, the Wadsworth VA Hospital in Los Angeles, and Oxford, England. Even the august premises of the *New York Times,* where some of the research for this chapter was performed, has not been immune. An outbreak of at least half a dozen cases occurred there in July of 1985.

It is now recognized that *Legionella* is a rather ubiquitous organism, and, through either epidemic outbreaks or sporadic cases in individuals, it accounts for an estimated fifty thousand cases annually of pneumonia in the United States alone (2 percent of all pneumonias in the nation). It is likely to be present in warm water all over the world. In industrialized countries, air conditioning systems are a frequent source. Whenever proper conditions for growth, aerosolization, and dispersion occur among susceptible individuals, an outbreak is likely to result. In Pontiac, although they never recovered the organism, the air conditioners were clearly implicated. Guinea pigs that inhaled an aerosol prepared from the water from the cooling towers developed the disease. No bacteria were recovered from the water samples collected from the air conditioner system at Bellevue Stratford, but this was most likely due to them having died off before they could be properly cultured.

Fortunately, the pneumonia resulting from *Legionella* infection is easily cured with the help of standard antibiotics, but many questions still remain. What accounts for the differing patterns of the disease? Pontiac fever was a relatively mild disease, with recovery uneventful and no deaths reported. In Philadelphia, one of six who came down with the disease died from it. Yet, as well as can be determined, the patients were infected with the same organism. Another epidemiological puzzle is why, with the organism so widely spread, will seemingly identical conditions give rise to an outbreak in one vicinity and not another?

More important than the lingering questions, perhaps, is the insight this episode has given us into the unending challenge that our microbial environment still presents to us. In modern societies at least, we tend to downgrade infectious diseases as being under control. We emphasize the "major killers," coronary heart disease and other complications of atherosclerosis as well as the threat of cancer. Yet microorganisms continue to deceive us with their seemingly unlimited capacity to disguise or mutate themselves into previously unrecognized human maladies. For example, even the common staphylococcus was able to develop a new twist and appear as the toxic shock syndrome. And now, infinitely more menacing, are the thousands upon thousands of new cases of AIDS, a viral infection attacking the immunological system.

What has happened to the principals of this tale more than a decade after the summer of 1976?

David Fraser's preoccupation with Legionnaire's disease in part gave his wife the opportunity to study law. As he moved up the bureaucratic ladder at CDC, she completed her education. When his wife was offered a promising position with the Securities and Exchange Commission in Washington, Fraser moved with her, assuming a new post as medical consultant with the Office of the Management of the Budget. Increasingly, his interest focused on education, and his activities as a Haverford alumnus expanded. At OMB, the head of the health branch turned out to be a Swarthmore alumnus. When Swarthmore was looking for a new executive, he placed Fraser's name in for consideration. Since 1982, as president of Swarthmore he has been able to indulge his interest in educational affairs, seeking ways to enhance the "ability to organize informational chaos in some systematic way."

Joseph McDade worked intensively on *Legionella* for about two years and then turned to other problems confronting him at CDC. He is now associate director for laboratory science at the Center for Infectious Diseases, a subdivision of the CDC. His new office boasts not one but three windows on the outer world, which includes a lovely view of downtown Atlanta.

Finally, the Bellevue-Stratford, two years after the debacle of 1976, was back in business, while *Legionella*, from what we now know of it, is unlikely ever to be out of it.

On Chinese Restaurants, Prolapsed Heart Valves, and Other Medical Conundrums

Medicine has been codified through centuries of observation and practice into groups of recognized diseases. They have been neatly grouped according to organ system and/or cause. Anything else with which we are confronted, unless it carries with it rather spectacular manifestations that simply cannot be ignored, is often dismissed as trivial, imaginary, or both. The "new" syndromes one reads about in the medical journals are often new only in the sense of being recently recognized officially and probably have been with us all along. However, thus documented, they now become respectable and are legitimized by a name.

"Ah yes, Mrs. Jones. You are suffering from Acute Idiopathic Cervicospinal Myalgia. I was just reading about it the other day . . ." (Translation: "Yes, I believe that you really do experience sudden pains in the muscles of your neck and upper back, although we have no idea of the cause—that is, idiopathic—but some respected authority has just reported ten cases of it in the latest edition of the *Annals of Internal Medicine*.") Functional hypoglycemia, mitral valve prolapse, and the Chinese Restaurant Syndrome all provide interesting examples of newly recognized syndromes that have provided reassurances to patients as well as their physicians.

The disorder now commonly called reactive or functional hypoglycemia was described originally in 1924 by Dr. Seale Harris of Birmingham, Alabama, but really began to catch on with the medical profession and the general public in the 1950s and 1960s.[1] The theory was that after a meal, some patients continued releasing insulin for hours, leading to drops in blood sugar levels and the manifestations of what might happen in any diabetic patient who has taken too much medication: an insulin reaction. These symptoms of palpitations, tingling, sweating, and nervousness also happen to describe an easily recognized psychiatric disorder, the typical "anxiety attack."

Inasmuch as anxiety attacks were recognized long before those of functional hypoglycemia became popularized, for many years possibly hypoglycemic patients were classified simply as slightly unbalanced mentally by their physicians. When functional hypoglycemia achieved recognition, many were suddenly removed from the looney category (as they and their friends would have considered any mental derangement, no matter how minor to their psychiatrists), and comfortably installed in the realm of endocrinology. So comfortable for the patients and convenient for their doctors was "functional hypoglycemia" that it became the frequent diagnosis for many puzzling complaints about which patients and their doctors knew next to nothing as to cause or cure. For those, patients and doctors alike, still convinced of this connection, recent evidence indicates that low blood sugars are most unlikely to be the cause of such symptoms following meals.[2]

In more recent times, mitral valve prolapse has come to supersede functional hypoglycemia as a favorite unsubstantiated diagnosis in patients with nagging but unexplainable symptomatology. Although systolic bulging of the mitral leaflets into the left atrium may be an accompaniment to other specific underlying heart diseases, it can exist as an isolated phenomenon rarely serious in nature, most often simply a normal variant with or without accompanying cardiac symptoms.

The mitral prolapse story has gone through several phases. For years, certain clicking sounds or murmurs heard in patients were thought by their doctors to be on an extracardiac basis (that is, due to minor abnormalities of other chest structures). Then, thanks to three South Africans, the true cause of these phenomena became apparent. In 1961, Dr. J. V. Reid revived the concept that such clicks/murmurs arose in the heart, and then, through the clinical and angiographic study of large numbers of such patients, Drs. John Barlow and Wendy Pocock demonstrated that the cause for such findings was the mitral valve pattern of motion.[3]

It was the advent of echocardiography, however, that really put mitral prolapse "on the map," especially with the growing realization that angiographic studies were often subject to unacceptable variability in interpretation. Now, with a simple, noninvasive technique, the diagnosis could be made easily, especially in asymptomatic individuals or those with symptoms so minor as not to warrant cardiac catheterization to establish the diagnosis. In those patients with marked symptomatology suggestive of heart disease—and they ran the gamut from palpitations to chest pain to fatigue and dizziness—doctors finally had an explanation of the symptoms and were able to convince their patients and themselves that the symptoms were not simply imaginary. Furthermore, in almost all cases doctors could assure the patients that, whatever the severity of their symptoms, their long-term outlook was excellent.

Then, gradually, confusion crept into the picture. First, it became recognized that some symptomatic patients with mitral prolapse on echocardiography did not have the telltale click/murmurs when physicians listened to their hearts ("silent prolapse"). Even early on, with the ready availability and ease of cardiac ultrasound, prevalence studies in the general population revealed that many asymptomatic normals, especially young women, could demonstrate prolapse on echocardiography. From this, physicians learned that mitral prolapse in many individuals was simply a normal variant of heart structure. Finally, even the symptoms of mitral prolapse were deprived of their validity: studies of patients with and without mitral prolapse on echocardiography now suggest no difference in the incidence of most if not all of the symptoms once considered typical of the syndrome.

Even the echocardiographic diagnosis of the prolapse

pattern has undergone significant evolution. The earliest technique, M-mode, missed some cases, which were then diagnosed by two-dimensional echocardiography, a later development. Then it was recognized that some of the 2-D criteria had been too loosely applied: many subjects had been labeled as having prolapse when the pattern this was based on, in certain views, was simply due to the normal variation of the pattern of valve insertion. As far as echocardiography is concerned, revisionism has reached such a point that in some quarters the criteria for a diagnosis of prolapse have become so restrictive that even patients with obvious click/murmurs—whom most doctors would accept as having prolapse—are now being denied the diagnosis by these investigators.

This is all very unfortunate because, in my view, there may be much more harm in underdiagnosing the condition than in granting it to patients in distress. The prognosis is almost invariably excellent, and thus reassuring to both doctor and patient. Furthermore, the medications prescribed for it, beta blockers, are often effective and reasonably safe. Their toning down of sympathetic discharges, whatever the cause, can be very helpful and if used only in times of stress can sustain the patients quite effectively over the long haul. (Many are the medical students I have helped through exam time with the judicious use of this diagnosis and treatment!)

The so-called Chinese Restaurant Syndrome provides a somewhat different kind of paradigm, but one that struck quite close to home for me. For years my sister-in-law complained about some ill-defined strange feelings each time she emerged from certain Chinese restaurants. These symptoms were experienced by no one else who accompanied her. As for the cause of her distress, we felt that she was an otherwise perfectly delightful, dependable, and reasonable member of the family and certainly entitled to this one strange quirk. Then in April of 1968 a physician, appropriately named Kwok, wrote a letter to the editor of the *New England Journal of Medicine*.[4] In it he described a peculiar set of symptoms: a numbness or tingling at the back of the neck that extended over the shoulders and either down the arms or into the chest with a tight feeling about the temples. They only occurred fifteen to twenty minutes after he had completed eating dinner, usually Mandarin style, at one or two Chinese restaurants he frequented. He wondered whether anyone else had knowledge of this disorder inasmuch as he had searched the medical literature for a description but to no avail.

In the ensuing weeks almost a dozen physicians and medical students had their letters printed in the journal. They too had suffered similar symptoms under the same circumstances. Their sense of relief in finding a fellow sufferer, and knowing that it was not "just in the head," was obvious. Since then, numerous more systematic forays into the mysteries of the syndrome have been made. Monosodium glutamate, used to enhance flavor, turns out to be the likely culprit. But, whatever the cause, it is now a perfectly respectable disorder with which to be afflicted.

The desire for symptomatic patients to be granted the sanctuary of a syndrome is probably matched only by the desire of certain intrepid or ambitious physicians to invent new ones to accommodate them. Failing this, they cannot resist the temptation of attempting publication of reports that can only be classified in the category of "Can you top this?" They may not raise the curtain on a new era of medical science, but at least they may raise a few eyebrows in the medical community.

One of the most common complaints among the general public, for example, is "gas," but it never really has received the kind of attention it might conceivably merit. An exception to this exclusion of serious scientific concern came ten years ago when "Studies of a flatulent patient" were performed by a team at the University of Minnesota and published in the *New England Journal of Medicine*, of all places.[5] Before arriving at that fount of knowledge in the heart of Minneapolis, a twenty-eight-year-old man had consulted seven different physicians about his complaint. None of them had had anything to offer, and the patient had been reduced to keeping his own "flatographic" records. Over a one-year period, it was later determined by statistical analysis that he passed flatus an average of 34 ± 7.3 (standard deviation) times a day.

Under the meticulous observation of the Minnesota group, the patient was encouraged to continue his accurate record keeping. For their part, his physicians analyzed the gas and at one point even collected it to determine volume. (The methodology for the latter was not described, but it certainly provided an exercise for the imagination.) Finally, with the help of a lactose-free diet, the daily gas-pass rate was reduced to 25 ± 8.2 S.D., a significant drop from the number of daily episodes he came in with. The authors were not totally immune to the potential responses of their readership. They concluded:

"At present, the patient is assiduously testing a variety of foods in an attempt to develop a flatus-free palatable diet— thus far without a whiff of success."

His experience with the University of Minnesota could not have been a total loss for the young man with the billowing bowels. There is always what the psychiatrists like to call "secondary gain" in conditions of adversity. During the course of his dietary manipulations, the effect of milk—two liters per day for two days—was observed. The result was an incredible daily flatus frequency of 141, with seventy passages in one four-hour period. This was submitted to the *Guinness Book of World Records* in hopeful anticipation.

Another investigator, this time from the Cleveland Clinic, has published an article entitled "ACHOO Syndrome" which means exactly how it sounds.[6] He reported that four of twenty neurologists questioned after a grand rounds conference held by the department admitted to sneezing when gazing into a bright light. Since I have been doing this myself all my life, I took the trouble to question fifty randomly selected individuals passing me in the hallways of my own institution. After overcoming certain feelings of apprehension about my mental state, twelve people, or 24 percent of the total, admitted to a similar pattern of photic response. Now, to save you countless sleepless nights pondering the meaning of all this, the author of this epic-making discovery has deduced that the cause lies not in our stars, dear reader, but in our genes. Believe it or not, the photic reflex may actually be an autosomal dominant with variable expressivity.

A team of researchers from Boston's Brigham-Women's Hospital have demonstrated even more enviable chutzpah in their description of two cases of "Giggle Incontinence."[7] Anyone who has ever heard of the expression "I laughed so hard the tears ran down my leg" can certainly appreciate that one!

And for all philanderers, a ready source of comfort has been on tap for years in a letter to the editor of the *New England Journal of Medicine* again. It describes "Sexual Intercourse and Transient Global Amnesia" in two patients. The next time your dalliance is suspected, simply reply, "What motel? What intercourse?" and refer to the April 12, 1979, issue.

What other fascinating ailments are awaiting the attention of some totally honest but foolhardy physician? The "Chronic Fatigue Syndrome" certainly looms on the horizon as a likely contender, whatever its relationship to the Epstein-Barr virus.[8] Certainly there are millions of us who are chronically fatigued and would love to be able to blame it on some "bug." For my part, however, since the strict scholarly category is disclaimed here, there is no hesitation in putting forth my own prime candidate: The Cine-cephalgia Galoshes Syndrome.

As a child, en route to a Saturday movie matinee on a rainy afternoon, I was frequently admonished by my mother to remove my galoshes in the theater or else suffer a severe headache and premature blindness. To this day, the neglect of this ritual in a darkened motion picture house results in a troublesome pain behind the eyes and a slight blurring of vision. One day I laughingly recounted this to a friend and his mother. The latter quickly replied, "Of course, everybody knows that!" We now await a high-powered team of experts from the National Institutes of Health to report on the effects of rubber-enclosed extremities on reflex pathways between the sensory receptors of the toes and certain regions of the brain.

Epilogue
Unfinished Business

"When in 1903, I began to look for a research problem in the field of circulation, I could not cull from the literature any significant problem that either remained unsolved or seemed solvable by available tools; the cream seemed to have been skimmed off in the nineteenth century."

—Carl J. Wiggers, 1960

As a young physician embarking on a career in cardiovascular research and practice, I soon became aware of the name of Dr. Carl J. Wiggers (1883–1963). Initially trained as a medical doctor, he already was at work on cardiovascular research as a medical student at the University of Michigan and, upon graduation, naturally gravitated into the department of physiology. He decided against going into the practice of clinical medicine and eventually ended up at Western Reserve in Cleveland, where he headed the Department of Physiology and spent the bulk of his professional life from 1918 to the time of his retirement in 1953.

During the thirty-five years at Western Reserve, he established a record of excellence and productivity that has been unequaled in the field of circulation at any other department in this country. Perhaps his greatest contribution, however, was the training of new investigators for cardiovascular research. Thirty-seven of his professional heirs went on to become departmental chairmen or directors of major research institutes. By the early 1960s, when I began my own work in the field, the names of graduates from his program read like a who's who of American circulatory physiology.

I found Wiggers's autobiography inspiring, and it became my personal primer as I took my own first tentative steps in cardiovascular research.[1] It was a later writing of Dr. Wiggers, however, from which I have derived the most enduring and inspiring message. The quoted lines are from an article he wrote for the *Bulletin of Medical History* as an introduction to a set of essays on various aspects of achievement in cardiovascular research over the previous century.[2] Framed, the quote has hung on the wall of my office for more than twenty-five years, a reminder to me as well as my trainees that, no matter how far we have come, no matter how neatly the answers seem to have fallen into place, no matter how impossible it may seem to achieve any further progress—there is always more work to be done.

At the time the young Wiggers was despairing of any meaningful research to perform in the field of the circulatory system, we were awaiting the recognition of the importance of hypertension and coronary heart disease as major health hazards; also the use of cardiac catheterization and angiographic techniques for the diagnosis of heart disease. A virtual explosion of new drugs for the treatment of heart disease was about to take place. The cardiac defibrillator would help cut in half the number of deaths from acute myocardial infarction and enable restoration of normal cardiac rhythm under a variety of other circumstances. Cardiac surgery would become a routine procedure, first without the use of cardiopulmonary bypass and then with the pump, enabling open-heart correction of a multiplicity of defects, including the insertion of artificial valves. Temporary and permanent cardiac pacemaking would prolong innumerable lives.

In fields unrelated to cardiology, other leaps of progress were in the offing. Antibiotics, the discovery of insulin, DNA, electron microscopy, kidney dialysis, to mention but a few. We would find it possible to transplant some organs and develop the ability to detect to a billionth of a gram the secretions of others. Artificial ears, joints, limbs, and eye parts would become part of our medical armamentarium. We would find better ways of preventing unwanted births and, for those with fertility problems, find ways of "growing babies in test tubes."

Not a bad record over less than a hundred years. But there is the other side of the coin.

With the development of microbiology in the late nineteenth century, the growth of immunology, and the introduction of the sulfa drugs, penicillin, and their progeny, the conquest of infectious disease seemed a real possibility in the 1940s and 1950s. True, smallpox has been completely eliminated, a wonderful achievement, and polio, at least in developed countries, has been brought under control. But other diseases once suppressed are now seriously on the rise and, added to these, are totally new infections to plague us.

The spread of malaria, initially reduced by DDT and other public health measures, has had over a twofold increase in worldwide prevalence over the last twenty to thirty years. With hundreds of millions of new cases each year and an annual mortality rate of about a million in Africa alone, it remains perhaps the most devastating disease on the planet. Its control has been further complicated by the emergence of strains resistant to the medications that have ordinarily been prescribed for it in the past. Another parasitic disease, schistosomiasis, is only somewhat less a threat, affecting 200 million people throughout the world and accounting for about 800,000 deaths annually. Tuberculosis still accounts for over a million deaths annually. Despite effective means of immunization, millions of third world infants and children continue to die each year from measles, whooping cough, and tetanus.

Although more developed societies in more temperate zones may not be threatened by such diseases as malaria and schistosomiasis, there are other ample causes for concern about infectious disease. Sexually transmitted diseases continue to constitute a major health problem, fueled in no small part by the use of intravenous drugs, the sale of sex for drugs, and a variety of sexual practices. Syphilis is on the rise; gonorrhea, increasingly in forms resistant to traditional antibiotics, continues a common health concern. Resistant forms of tuberculosis are also being encountered now with increasing frequency.

Among newly recognized diseases with which to contend, venereal infections such as genital herpes, chlamydia, and papilloma virus probably account for more than five million cases a year in the United States alone. *Legionella* and Lyme disease have entered into the ordinary differential diagnosis of infections, and, most ominous of all, AIDS has arrived to present a major health threat throughout the world.

We are not doing too well with cancer despite all the knowledge we have gained about the process.[3] Mortality from cancer has risen rather than declined over the last thirty years. While spectacular progress has been made in the treatment of some childhood cancers, with true cures achieved for previously rapidly fatal leukemias, for example, these constitute only a small fraction of all cancers among the population. In lung cancer, still number one among adult malignancies, there is no real improvement. In breast cancer, we have seen the end to mutilating surgery and perhaps a few more patients than before are being saved by early diagnosis. Overall, however, the improvement, if any, has not been dramatic, and one in every ten or eleven American women living to the age of sixty-five can expect to develop it. Only in colon cancer has some increase in survival been shown, perhaps because of earlier diagnosis and treatment. The diagnosis of esophageal or pancreatic cancers remains essentially an early death warrant.

The aging of the population presents new challenges. Debilitating and enormously costly illnesses of the aged are straining the health care system. Strokes, Alzheimer's disease, and Parkinsonism are all preeminent problems among the elderly, without even venturing outside the nervous system. These and other health concerns of a population in the United States that will consist of 20 percent of people sixty-five or over by 2020 have not been adequately addressed.

Public health experts have pointed out that over the past century better nutrition, better living conditions, and sanitary improvements, along with social progress, have been responsible in large part for improvements in health. Yet today technology seems to be working against the public good. We seem to be at war with our environment, polluting the air, contaminating once pristine rivers and streams, and denuding once luxuriant forests. Industrialization seems to be running amok, with places like the Love Canal, Bhopal, and Chernobyl chilling reminders of our ecological ineptitude.

We are deluged with problems of population. We have devised effective methods of birth control so that the planet can support its future inhabitants, but we cannot implement them effectively. Even under so oppressive and dominating regime as that of Communist China, the urge to procreate cannot be contained. The policy of "One family, one child" has failed miserably, and in 1989, there were 1.1 billion mouths to feed. With 20 percent of the world's population and only 7 percent of its arable land, China can only hope that the arrival of the next 100 million can be slowed somewhat.

Elsewhere in the world, we strive to decrease infant mortality with vaccines and public health measures only to see the same children starve as a result of mismanagement of land and water resources, changing climate, and political considerations that make drought and starvation an ever present threat.

Indeed, there is still much work that remains to be done. But, despite the gloomy picture I have drawn, there is reason to believe that new technology, new people, new ideas, and new discoveries will manage to brighten it.

As microbiology led to progress in the nineteenth century, molecular biology and continued advances in immunology hold out hope for the twentieth. Aided by advances in electronics, chemistry, and computer science, these may well lead to the next great leap forward in understanding and treating a variety of human ailments.

We have already witnessed how recombinant DNA technology has permitted the production of synthetic insulin and growth hormone, among other important biological substances. The mapping of the human gene will, no doubt, provide important insights into the management of many important diseases that have been shown to have genetic components. Many insulin-dependent diabetics, Alzheimer's disease sufferers, those with cystic fibrosis, manic-depressives, and many cancer patients may one day profit from this type of research. Does gene replacement or modification in the cure of such patients seem any more farfetched in 1990 than kidney and heart transplantation did in 1950?

In the field of immunology, the ability to produce monoclonal antibodies is more than a research tool. The technique may one day be used routinely to track cancer cells and even eliminate them in instances where surgical, chemical, and radiation techniques have failed. Newer vaccines are being developed for the prevention of malaria, schistosomiasis, and even for the human immunodeficiency virus, the cause of AIDS. The hepatitis B virus, endemic in certain parts of the world, has been linked to primary liver cancer, a major cause of death among relatively young people in Asia and Africa. The use of immunological techniques already available has been shown in several third world countries to reduce the incidence of chronic hepatitis in infants born to infected mothers. It is hoped that treatment of these newborns will also reduce the later development of primary liver cancer in this population.

A strong pharmaceutical industry is essential to the development of new drugs. Oftentimes it is only they, rather than some governmental agency, that can invest the money and resources into a line of research that promises to produce the next "wonder drug" or capitalize on investigating an agent that has demonstrated serendipitously a totally unanticipated type of biological effect. There seems to be no diminishment of effort on the part of this important resource here and abroad.

AIDS, for all its horrific aspects, provides a paradigm of what modern science can accomplish. Compare its history, comprising only a little more than a decade, with that of poliomyelitis. Over the past ten years, we have learned more about the cause, transmission, prevention, and even treatment of AIDS than we did in more than a hundred years of study with polio. It is something of which modern science can be proud.

Beyond the boundaries of the laboratories and the clinics, there is added encouragement to be gained from a growing awareness on the part of our governments of the roles they must play in the preservation of our health. Mechanisms and agencies are in place, even though they are not always employed vigorously. For the first time, in 1989, an international conference convened to discuss the problems of pollution and global warming. A decrease in tensions between the United States and the Soviet Union promises a lessening interest in the building up of nuclear arms and a new emphasis on recognizing the hazards of nuclear waste.

A rising awareness of our citizenry is also apparent. We know that many of our illnesses are self-induced. Antismoking campaigns have shown success. We are beginning to hold our politicians responsible for their actions as they affect our environment.

All this is encouraging, but, as the stories in this book demonstrate, the pathways to discovery are often individual and unexpected. In addition to planned research, we must always be receptive to such unusual sources of progress. In his recent autobiography, Nobelist François Jacob makes many cogent remarks about the unpredictability of science: "Late, very late, I discovered the true nature of science, of how it proceeds, of the men who do it. I came to understand that, contrary to what I believed, the march of science does not consist in a series of inevitable conquests, or advance along the royal road of human reason, or result necessarily and inevitably from conclusive observations dictated by experimentation and argument."[4]

Later on, Jacob contrasts "day science" and "night science." The first "employs reasoning that meshes like gears, and achieves results with the force of certainty." The second is characterized as wandering blindly, hazy, proceeding along sinuous streets and blind alleys. It is likened to a prisoner in a cell "looking for a way out, a glimmer of light."[5]

This remark of Jacob's reminded me of another's, in a rather different context but nonetheless apt. Adlai Stevenson paraphrased the motto of a religious organization, the Christophers, in eulogizing a great lady, Eleanor Roosevelt. The original quotation goes: Better to light one candle than to curse the darkness.

Given the tasks before us, could any of us disagree?

Notes

Mercury Finally "Makes It"

1. An excellent detailed history of mercury and medicine is Leonard J. Goldwater's *Mercury: A History of Quicksilver* (Baltimore: York Press, 1972).

2. Cellini's cure was deduced by surgeon Glenn W. Geelhoed (*Australia and New Zealand Journal of Surgery* 48 (1978): 589–594).

3. Walter Pagee, "Paracelsus," in *Dictionary of Scientific Biography*, vol. 10. ed. Charles C. Gillispie (New York: Scribner's, 1974), 304–313.

4. J. Addison Freeman, "Mercurial disease among hatters," *Transactions of the Medical Society of New Jersey* (1860): 61–64.

5. Alfred Vogl, "The discovery of the organic mercurial diuretics," *American Heart Journal* 39 (1950): 881–883.

6. Paul Saxl and Robert Heilig, "Über die diuretische Wirkung von novasural—und angeren Quecksilberinjektionen," *Wien Clin Wchnschr* 33 (1920): 943–945.

7. William Dock in Allen B. Weisse, *Conversations in Medicine. The Story of Twentieth-Century American Medicine in the Words of Those Who Created It* (New York: New York University Press, 1984), 20.

Why Do They Turn Yellow?
The Centuries-long Search for the Viruses of Hepatitis

1. For an excellent up-to-date history of all developments in the study of liver disease, see Thomas S. Chen and Peter S. Chen, *Understanding the Liver. A History* (Westport Conn: Greenwood Press, 1984).

2. Much of the material related to these three men was obtained through personal interviews conducted on March 19, 1987 in New York City (Dr. Prince); March 30, 1987 in New York City (Dr. Krugman); and May 30, 1987 in Philadelphia (Dr. Blumberg). These and all subsequent interviews conducted for this book were first recorded on tape. The narratives derived therefrom and constituting major portions of the individual chapters were

sent to each of the principals for corrections, additions, and so forth, before being submitted for publication in final form.

3. E. A. Cockayne, "Catarrhal jaundice, sporadic and epidemic, and its relation to acute yellow atrophy of the liver," *Quart J Med* 6 (1912): 1–29.

4. S. Krugman, J. P. Giles, and J. Hammond, "Infectious hepatitis. Evidence for two distinctive clinical, epidemiological and immunological types of infection," *JAMA* 200 (1967): 365–373.

5. A. M. Prince, H. Fuji, and R. K. Gershon, "Immunohistochemical studies on the etiology of anicteric hepatitis in Korea." *Am J Hyg* 79 (1964): 365–381.

6. B. S. Blumberg, H. J. Alter, and S. Visnich, "A 'new' antigen in leukemia sera," *JAMA* 191 (1965): 541–546.

7. In an article published in 1967 (B. S. Blumberg, B. J. S. Gerstley, D. A. Hungerford, et al., "A serum antigen (Australia antigen) in Down's Syndrome, leukemia and hepatitis," *Annals Int Med* 66 [1967]: 924–931), Blumberg and his coworkers concluded, "Most of the disease associations *could* [italics added] be explained by the association of Au with a virus, as suggested in our previous publications."

Prince's more forceful interpretation of the results of their collaboration was stated in a letter to the editor of *Lancet* (A. M. Prince, "Relation of Australia antigen and SH antigens," *Lancet* 2 [1968]: 462–463): "In conclusion, these findings suggest that Australia antigen and SH (serum hepatitis) antigen are closely related, and perhaps identical."

8. D. S. Dane, C. H. Cameron and M. Briggs, "Virus-like particles in serum of patients with Australia-antigen-associated hepatitis," *Lancet* 1 (1970): 695–698.

9. S. Krugman, J. P. Giles, and J. Hammond, "Hepatitis virus. Effect of heat on the infectivity and antigenicity of the MS-1 and MS-2 strains," *J Infect Dis* 122 (1970): 432–436.

10. Letter from Dr. Maurice R. Hilleman dated June 23, 1987. The Hilleman and Blumberg accounts of the hepatitis B vaccine development are somewhat at odds with each other. I have tried to be as objective as possible in relating these events.

11. W. Szmuness, C. E. Stevens, E. J. Harley, et al., "Hepatitis B vaccine. Demonstration of efficacy in a controlled clinical trial in a high risk population in the United States," *New Engl J Med* 303 (1980): 833–841.

12. J. P. Giles, "Hepatitis research among retarded children," *Lancet* 1 (1971): 1126. More recently, Dr. Krugman has written about this whole question in retrospect (S. Krugman, "The Willowbrook hepatitis studies revisited: Ethical aspects," *Rev Inf Dis* 8 (1986): 157–162.

Into the Heart
The Surgical Treatment of Heart Disease Becomes a Reality

1. H. Engle, "Billroth, Christian Albert Theodor," in *Dictionary of Scientific Biography*, vol 2, ed. C. C Gillispie (New York: Scribner's, (1970): 129–131.

2. For years, Billroth was unjustly criticized for including this dictum as part of his published teaching regarding cardiac surgery. Rudolf Nissen, a German surgeon assisting the great Ernst Sauerbruch in the preparation of the second volume (1925) of his book on thoracic surgery, was assigned by his chief to trace the source of this statement. Nissen tracked down a surviving assistant of Billroth's, a Dr. von Eiselberg, who recalled Billroth making this remark in passing but not publishing it (R. Nissen, "Billroth and cardiac surgery [ltr]," *Lancet* 2 [1963]: 250–251). Searches by others to find this opinion in Billroth's papers and monographs have similarly failed to document this opposition to cardiac surgery as part of his official position on the subject.

3. F. B. Berry, Preface in *Surgery in World War II: Thoracic Surgery*, Vol 2 (Washington, D.C.: Office of the Surgeon General, Dept. of Army, 1965), xiii.

4. Among the books on the history of cardiac surgery that I have found especially useful are Robert G. Richardson, *The Scalpel and the Heart* (New York: Scribner's, 1970) and Stephen L. Johnson, *The History of Cardiac Surgery, 1896–1955* (Baltimore: Johns Hopkins Press, 1970). An excellent abbreviated history by Dr. Robert S. Litwak can be found in *Cardiovascular Clinics* ("The growth of cardiac surgery. Historical notes," *Cardiovasc Clin* Vol 3, no 2, guest ed. D. E. Harken, [1971]: 6–49).

5. J. Moseley, "Alexis Carrel. The man unknown," *JAMA* 244 (1980): 1119–1121; E. Bendiner, "The paradox of Alexis Carrel," *Hospital Practice* (Feb. 1981): 125–145.

6. Abbott's own recollections are contained in an "autobiographical sketch" (*McGill Med J* 28 [1959]: 127–152). For later evaluations of her contributions, see C. G. Roland, "Maude Abbott and J. B. MacCallum. Canadian cardiac pioneers," *Chest* 57 (1970): 371–377, and K. Smith, "Maude Abbott: pathologist and historian," *Canad Med Ass J* 127 (1982): 774–776.

7. Maude E. Abbott, *Atlas of Congenital Cardiac Disease* (New York: American Heart Association, 1936).

8. Taussig's recollections are contained in H. B. Taussig, "On the evolution of our knowledge of congenital malformations of the heart. The T. Duckett Jones Lecture," *Circulation* 31 (1965): 768–777, and H. B. Taussig, "Neuhauser Lecture. Tetralogy of Fallot: Early history and late results," *Am J Roent* 133 (1979): 423–431.

There is also an interview with Taussig on videotape by Dr. Helen S. Pittman, part of a series entitled "Leaders of American Medicine," National Medical Audiovisual Center in cooperation with Alpha Omega Alpha, 1974.

For some personal evaluations of her career (following her death in 1986), see J. A. Manning, M. A. Engle, R. Whittemore, C. A. Neill, and C. Ferencz, "Historical milestones: Helen Brooke Taussig: 1898–1986," *J Am Coll Card* 10 (1987): 662–671.

9. The first edition of her pioneering monograph on the subject appeared in 1947 (Helen B. Taussig, *Congenital Malformations of the Heart* [New York: Commonwealth Fund, 1947]). This was later revised for a second edition which appeared in 1960.

10. R. M. Marquis, "Congenital heart disease: the ductus arteriosus as pathfinder," *Br Heart J* 58 (1987): 429–436.

11. R. Warren, "Landmark perspective. Patent ductus arteriosus," *JAMA* 251 (1984): 1203–1207.

12. Two highly respected medical historians who reviewed the manuscript expressed doubts about the veracity of this story. By the time I began to probe into it, Dr. Gross was dead. Dr. Warren, who repeated the tale in his commentary on the landmark article reprinted in the *Journal of the American Medical Association*, had accepted it at face value. I then sought the assistance of several reliable senior physicians in the Boston area. None were able to uncover the name of the pediatrician or verify the incident. My conclusion is that although the story is probably apocryphal, Dr. Gross believed it, repeated it, but never bothered to check it out for himself.

13. R. E. Gross, J. P. Hubbard, "Surgical ligation of a patent ductus arteriosus," *JAMA* 112 (1939): 729–731.

14. A. Blalock and H. B. Taussig, "The surgical treatment of malformations of the heart in which there is pulmonary stenosis or pulmonary atresia," *JAMA* 128 (1945): 182–202. Also see D. G. McNamara, "Landmark perspective. The Blalock-Taussig operation and subsequent progress in surgical treatment of cardiovascular diseases," *JAMA* 251 (1984): 2139–2141.

15. C. Crafoord and G. Nylin, "Congenital coarctation of the aorta and its surgical treatment," *J Thor Surg* 14 (1945): 347–361.

16. E. C. Cutler and S. A. Levine, "Cardiotomy and valvulotomy for mitral stenosis," *Boston Med J* 188 (1923): 1023–1027.

17. H. S. Souttar, "The surgical treatment of mitral stenosis," *Brit Med J* 2 (1925): 603–606.

18. Charles P. Bailey in Weisse, *Conversations in Medicine*, 133–156.

19. Gibbon recalled his experiences in two articles: J. H. Gibbon, Jr., "The gestation and birth of an idea," *Philadelphia Medicine* (Sept. 13, 1963): 913–916, and J. H. Gibbon, Jr., "The development of the heart-lung apparatus," *Am J Surg* 135 (1978): 608–619.

20. André Cournand in Weisse, *Conversations in Medicine*, 111–131.

21. J. H. Comroe, Jr., and R. D. Dripps, "Ben Franklin and open heart surgery," *Circ Res* 35 (1974): 661–669.

The Long Pause:
The Discovery and Rediscovery of Penicillin

1. Gwyn Macfarlane, *Alexander Fleming. The Man and the Myth* (Cambridge, Mass: Harvard University Press, 1984) and Gwyn Macfarlane, *Howard Florey. The Making of a Great Scientist* (Oxford: Oxford University Press, 1979).

2. R. Hare, "New light on the history of penicillin," *Med Hist* 26 (1982): 1–24.

3. Although this is the most popular version of the beginning of the penicillin story, it is not the only one. Variations on this and other aspects of the development of penicillin are discussed in detail in Milton Wainright's book *Miracle Cure* (Oxford: Blackwells, 1990).

4. A. Fleming, "On the antibacterial action of cultures of a Penicillium with special reference to their use in the isolation of B. influenzae," *Brit J Exp Path* 10 (1929): 226–236.

5. *Nobel Lectures. Physiology or Medicine. 1942–1962* Amsterdam, Elsevier, (1964): 83–145.

Turning Bad Luck into Good:
The Alchemy of Willem Kolff, the First Successful Artificial Kidney and the Artificial Heart

1. Much of the material herein is based on a personal interview with Dr. Kolff (Weisse, *Conversations in Medicine*, 342–373). Dr. Kolff has also published an account of his early experiences with the artificial kidney ("First clinical experience with the artificial kidney," *Ann Int Med* 62 [1965]: 608–619). Also see W. S. Kolff, "Past, present and future of artificial kidneys," *Transpl Proc* 13, suppl. 1 (1981): 35–40.

2. For an excellent review of the history of dialysis, see P. McBride, "The development of hemo- and peritoneal dialysis," in *Clinical Dialysis*, ed. A. R. Nissenson, R. N. Fine, and D. E. Gentile (Norwalk: Appleton-Century Crofts, 1984), 1–27.

3. J. J. Abel, L. G. Rountree, and B. B. Turner, "On the removal of diffusible substances from the circulating blood of living animals by dialysis," *J Pharm Exp Therap* 5 (1914): 275–316.

4. P. T. McBride, *Genesis of the Artificial Kidney* (Deerfield: Travenol Laboratories, 1979). An accompanying film, including rare film footage of Abel and Necheles plus interviews with many of the more recent principals, is available on loan from Travenol as well.

5. J. Benedum, "Georg Haas (1886–1971) Pionier der Hämodialyse," *Med Hist J* 14 (1979): 196–217.

6. Personal correspondence, Dr. W. Drukker of Amsterdam, July 22, 1987.

7. H. Popper, "In memoriam. Isadore Snapper, 1889–1973," *Mt Sinai J Med* 40 (1973): 716–719.

Say It Isn't "No":
The Power of Positive Thinking in the Publication of Medical Research

1. Julius H. Comroe, Jr., *Retrospectroscope. Insights into Medical Discovery* (Menlo Park: Von Gehr Press, 1977) and J. H. Comroe, Jr. and R. D. Dripps, "Ben Franklin and open heart surgery," *Circ Res* 35 (1974): 661–669.

2. J. Fibiger, "Recherches sur un nématode et sur sa faculté de provoquer des neoformations papillomateuses et carcinomateuses dans l'estomac du rat," *Acad Royale Sci Lettres Danemark* (1913): 1–41.

3. W. Wernstedt, Presentation speech in *Nobel Lectures: Physiology or Medicine, 1922–1941* (Amsterdam: Elsevier, 1965): 119–121.

4. P. Rous, "A sarcoma of the fowl transmissible by an agent separable from the tumor cells," *J Exp Med* 13 (1911): 397–411.

5. J. H. Tijo, and A. Levan, "The chromosome number in man," *Hereditas* 42 (1956): 1–6.

6. G. C. Cotzias, M. H. Van Woert, and L. M. Schliffer, "Aromatic amino acids and modification of parkinsonism," *New Engl J Med* 276 (1967): 374–379.

7. Leon J. Kamin, *The Science and Politics of IQ* (Potomac, Md: L. Erlbaum Assoc., 1974).

An Anemia Called "Pernicious"

1. For a biography of Whipple, see George W. Corner, *George Whipple and His Friends; the Life story of a Nobel Prize Pathologist* (Philadelphia: Lippincott, 1963).

2. W. B. Castle, "The contributions of George Richards Minot to experimental medicine," *New Engl J Med* 247 (1952): 585–592.

3. William Parry Murphy in Weisse, *Conversations in Medicine*, 61–77.

4. G. R. Minot, and W. P. Murphy, "Treatment of pernicious anemia by a special diet," *JAMA* 87 (1926): 470–476.

5. Castle published a number of papers lucidly describing the progress of his research. These culminated in W. B. Castle and T. H. Ham, "Observations on the etiologic relationship of achylia gastrica to pernicious anemia. V. Further evidence for the essential participation of extrinisic factor in hematopoietic responses to mixtures of beef muscle and gastric juice and to hog stomach mucosa," *JAMA* 107 (1936): 1456–1463.

From Trench Warfare to War on Cancer:
The Development of Chemotherapy for Malignant Disease

1. Quoted in Richard Thoumin, *The First World War* (New York: Putnam's Sons, 1964), 175.

2. E. B. Krumbhaar, and H. D. Krumbhaar, "The blood and bone marrow in yellow cross gas (mustard gas) poisoning," *J Med Res* 40 (1919): 497–507.

3. Alfred Gilman's personal account of these beginnings was published as "The initial clinical trial of nitrogen mustard," *Am J Surg* 105 (1963): 574–578.

For an overview of the development of chemotherapy for cancer up to more recent times, see C. G. Zubrod, "Historic milestones in curative chemotherapy," *Sem Oncology* 6 (1979): 490–505. For additional, more personal commentary by the same author, see C. G. Zubrod, "The cure of cancer by chemotherapy. The Fifth Myron Karon Memorial Lecture," *Med Ped Onc* 8 (1980): 107–114.

4. Gilman, "The initial clinical trial of nitrogen mustard."

5. L. S. Goodman, M. M. Wintrobe, W. Dameshek, et al., "Nitrogen mustard therapy. Use of methyl-bis (beta-chloroethyl) amine hydrochloride and tris (beta-chloroethyl) amine hydrochloride for Hodgkin's disease, lymphosarcoma, leukemia and certain allied and miscellaneous disorders," *JAMA* 132 (1946): 126–132.

6. S. Farber, L. K. Diamond, R. D. Mercer, et al., "Effect of chemotherapeutic agents on acute leukemia; folic acid antagonists," *Am J Dis Child* 77 (1949): 129–130.

7. B. Rosenberg, L. Van Camp, and T. Krigas, "Inhibition of cell division in Escherichia coli by electrolysis products from a platinum electrode," *Nature* 205 (1965): 698–699.

8. Gilman, "The initial clinical trial of nitrogen mustard."

Sparks: Life-Giving Electricity

1. Dr. Uhley kindly assisted me in recalling the details of this case as well as reviewing the other contents of this chapter and providing helpful suggestions.

2. S. Furman, and J. B. Schwedel, "An intracardiac pacemaker for Stokes-Adams seizures," *New Engl J Med* 261 (1959): 943–948.

3. L. A. Geddes, "A Short History of the Electrical Stimulation of Excitable Tissue," *Physiologist* 27, suppl (1984): 1–43. (An excellent review of the subject.)

4. H. B. Burchell, "A centennial note on Waller and the first human electrocardiogram," *Am J Card* 59 (1987): " 979–983. For more on Waller, also see "Augustus Désiré Waller (1856–1922)," in *Cardiac Classics*, ed. F. A.

Willius and T. E. Keys (St. Louis: C. V. Mosby, 1941), 654–661, which includes a reprint of his report, "A demonstration on man of electromotive changes accompanying the heart's beat," *J Physiol* 8 (1887): 229–234. Also: "Augustus D. Waller (Obituary)" *Brit Med J* 1 (1922): 458–459.

5. "Willem Einthoven (1860–1927)" in *Cardiac Classics*. This features an English translation of his paper (originally in German), "The galvanometric registration of the human electrocardiogram, likewise a review of the use of the capillary-electrometer in physiology," *Pfluger's Arch f d ges Physiol* 99 (1903): 472–480.

6. I. Ershler, "Willem Einthoven—the man," *Arch Int Med* 148 (1988): 453–455.

7. Both accounts are reproduced in Willius and Keys' *Cardiac Classics*.

8. An interview with Dr. Zoll on November 11, 1987 in Anaheim, California. I am also deeply indebted to Dr. Zoll for his review of the chapter, with many helpful corrections and suggestions.

9. A. S. Hyman, "Resuscitation of the stopped heart by intracardial therapy," *Arch Int Med* 50 (1932): 283–305.

10. Ibid.

11. J. C. Callaghan and W. G. Bigelow, "An electrical artificial pacemaker for standstill of the heart," *Annals Surg* 134 (1951): 8–17.

12. P. M. Zoll, "Resuscitation of the heart in ventricular standstill by external electric stimulation," *New Engl J Med* 247 (1952): 768–771.

13. P. M. Zoll, A. J. Linenthal, W. Gibson, et al., "Intravenous drug therapy of Stokes-Adams disease," *Circulation* 17 (1958): 325–339.

14. Å. Senning (discussion of paper by Stephenson et al.), *J Thor Cardiovasc Surg* 38 (1959): 639.

15. W. M. Chardack, A. A. Gage, and W. Greatbatch, "A transistorized, self-contained, implantable pacemaker for the long-term correction of complete heart block," *Surgery* 48 (1960): 643–654.

16. W. B. Kouwenhoven, "The development of the defibrillator," *Ann Int Med* 71 (1969): 449–458.

17. J. L. Prevost, and F. Batelli, "Quelques effets des décharges électriques sur le coeur des mammifères," *J Physiol Path Gen* 1 (1900): 40–52.

18. T. E. Driscol, O. D. Ratnoff and O. F. Nygaard, "The remarkable Dr. Abildgaard and countershock," *Ann Int Med* 83 (1975): 878–882.

19. N. L. Gurvich, and G. S. Yuniev, "Restoration of heart rhythm during fibrillation by a condenser discharge," *Am Rev Soviet Med* 4 (1947): 252–256.

20. C. S. Beck, W. H. Pritchard, and H. S. Feil, "Ventricular fibrillation of long duration abolished by electric shock," *JAMA* 135 (1947): (1947): 985–986.

21. P. M. Zoll, et al., "Termination of ventricular fibrillation in man by externally applied electric countershock," *New Engl J Med* 254 (1956): 727–732.

22. H. W. Day, "An intensive coronary care area," *Chest* 44 (1963): 423–427.

23. M. Mirowski, "The automatic implantable cardioverter-defibrillator: an overview," *J Am Coll Card* 6 (1985): 461–466.

Polio
The Not-So-Twentieth-Century Disease

1. The best and most complete history of poliomyelitis, from antiquity to the introduction of the Salk and Sabin vaccines, is by Dr. John R. Paul: *A History of Poliomyelitis* (New Haven: Yale University Press, 1971).

2. Much of Dr. Rivers's story and especially his involvement with Drs. Sabin and Salk as well as the National Foundation for Infantile Paralysis is included in Dr. Saul Benison's oral history (*Tom Rivers. Reflections of a Life in Medicine and Science* [Cambridge, Mass.: MIT Press, 1967]). All quotes by Dr. Rivers are from this volume.

3. S. Flexner, and P. A. Lewis, "The transmission of acute poliomyelitis to monkeys," *JAMA* 53 (1989): 1639–1640.

4. Interview with Dr. Sabin, Washington, D.C. on July 27, 1987.

5. A. B. Sabin, and A. M. Wright, "Acute ascending myelitis following a monkey bite, with the isolation of a virus capable of reproducing the disease," *J Exp Med* 59 (1934): 115–136.

6. A. B. Sabin, and R. Ward, "The natural history of human poliomyelitis. I. Distribution of virus in nervous and non-nervous tissues," *J Exp Med* 73 (1941): 771–793.

7. J. F. Enders, T. H. Weller, and F. C. Robbins, "Cultivation of the Lansing strain of poliomyelitis virus in cultures of various human embryonic tissues," *Science* 109 (1949): 85–87.

8. Weisse, *Conversations in Medicine*, 163.

9. J. R. Paul, and J. T. Riordan, "Observations on serological epidemiology. Antibodies to the Lansing strain of poliomyelitis virus in sera from Alaskan Eskimos," *Am J Hyg* 52 (1950): 202–212.

10. For much of the Salk story, see Richard Carter, *Breakthrough: The Saga of Jonas Salk* (New York: Trident Press, 1966). This was supplemented and updated by a personal interview at the Salk Institute in La Jolla, California, on November 20, 1987. Direct quotes of Dr. Salk are from this interview.

11. T. Francis, Jr., R. F. Korns, R. B. Voight, et al., "An evaluation of the 1954 poliomyelitis vaccine trials: Summary report," *Am J Pub Health* 45 (1955): 1–63.

12. S. Benison, "International medical cooperation. Dr. Albert Sabin, live poliovirus vaccine and the Soviets," *Bull Med Hist* 56 (1982): 460–483.

13. A. M. McBean, and J. F. Modlin, "Rationale for the sequential use of

inactivated poliovirus vaccine and live attenuated poliovirus vaccine for routine poliomyelitis immunization in the United States," *Ped Inf Dis J* 6 (1987): 881–887.

Of Birds and Blood Cells:
Bruce Glick Unravels the Secret of the Bursa of Fabricius

1. Interview with Dr. Glick, Margate, New Jersey, in August 1986.

2. B. Zanobio, "Fabrici, Girolamo," in *Dictionary of Scientific Biography*, vol 4, ed. C. C. Gillespie (New York: Scribner's, 1971), 507–512.

3. B. Glick, T. S. Chang, and R. G. Jaap, "The bursa of Fabricius and antibody production," *Poultry Sci* 35 (1956): 224–225. Also see B. Glick, "Bursa of Fabricius," in *Avian Biology*, vol 7, ed. D. S. Farner et al. (San Diego: Academic Press, 1983): 443–500.

4. Robert A. Good in Weisse, *Conversations in Medicine*, 309–341. Also see R. A. Good, "Historical aspects of cellular immunology," in *Advances in Host Defense Mechanisms*, vol. 2, ed A. S. Fauci, and J. I. Gallin (New York: Raven Press, 1982).

5. Weisse, *Conversations in Medicine*, 323.

A Plague in Philadelphia:
The Story of Legionnaires' Disease

1. This chapter is based primarily on interviews with Dr. Joseph E. McDade (Atlanta, Georgia, on March 12, 1986) and Dr. David W. Fraser (Swarthmore, Pennsylvania, on June 20, 1986).

2. D. W. Fraser, T. R. Tsai, W. Orenstein, et al., "Legionnaires' Disease. Description of an epidemic of pneumonia," *New Engl J Med* 297 (1977): 1189–1197; J. E. McDade, C. C. Shepard, D. W. Fraser et al., "Legionnaires' Disease. Isolation of a bacterium and demonstration of its role in other respiratory disease," *New Engl J Med* 297 (1977): 1197–1203; and F. W. Chandler, M. D. Hicklin, and J. A Blackmon, "Demonstration of the agent of Legionnaires' Disease in tissue," *New Engl J Med* 297 (1977): 1218–1220.

3. "International Symposium on Legionnaires' Disease," ed. A. Balows, and D. W. Fraser, *Ann Int Med* 90 (1979): 491–707.

On Chinese Restaurants, Prolapsed Heart Valves, and Other Medical Conundrums

1. F. D. Hofeldt, "Reactive hypoglycemia," *Metabolism* 24 (1975): 1193–1208.

2. J. Palardy, J. Havrankova, R. LePage, et al., "Blood glucose measurements during symptomatic episodes in patients with suspected postprandial hypoglycemia," *New Engl J Med* 321 (1989): 1421–1425.

3. J. B. Barlow, and W. A. Pocock, "The problem of non-ejection systolic clicks and associated mitral systolic murmurs: Emphasis on the billowing mitral leaflet syndrome," *Am Heart J* 90 (1975): 636–655.

4. R. H. M. Kwok, "Chinese restaurant syndrome," *New Engl J Med* 278 (1968): 796.

5. M. D. Levitt, R. B Lasser, J. S. Schwartz, and J. H. Bond, "Studies of a flatulent patient," *New Engl J Med* 295 (1976): 260–262.

6. H. H. Morris, III, "ACHOO Syndrome," *Cleveland Clin J Med* 54 (1987): 431–433.

7. M. P. Rogers, R. F. Gittes, D. M. Dawson, and P. Reich, "Giggle incontinence," *JAMA* 247 (1982): 1446–1448.

8. G. P. Holmes, J. E Kaplan, N. M. Gantz, et al., "Chronic fatigue syndrome. A working case definition," *Ann Int Med* 108 (1988): 387–389.

Unfinished Business

1. Carl J. Wiggers, *Reminiscences and Adventures in Circulation Research* (New York: Grune and Stratton, 1958).

2. C. J. Wiggers, "Some significant advances in cardiac physiology during the nineteenth century," *Bull Hist Med* 34 (1960): 1–15.

3. J. C. Bailar III, and E. M. Smith, "Progress against cancer?," *New Engl J Med* 314 (1986): 1226–1232.

4. François Jacob, *The Statue Within* (New York: Basic Books, 1988), 8.

5. Ibid., 296.

Name Index

Subject Index